Clinician's Manual on Ankylosing Spondylitis

Joachim Sieper
Charité University Hospital
Campus Benjamin Franklin
Berlin, Germany

Jürgen Braun
Rheumatology Center Ruhrgeb
St Josefs Hospital
Herne, Germany

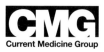

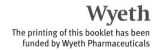
The printing of this booklet has been
funded by Wyeth Pharmaceuticals

Published by Current Medicine Group Ltd, 11–21 Paul Street, London EC2A 4JU, UK

www.currentmedicinegroup.com

Copyright © 2009 Current Medicine Group Ltd, a part of Springer Science+Business Media

ISBN 978-1- 85873-436-1

British Library Cataloguing-in-Publication Data.
A catalogue record for this book is available from the British Library.

Although every effort has been made to ensure that drug doses and other information are presented accurately in this publication, the ultimate responsibility rests with the prescribing physician. Neither the publishers nor the author can be held responsible for errors or for any consequences arising from the use of information contained herein. Any product mentioned in this publication should be used in accordance with the prescribing information prepared by the manufacturers. No claims or endorsements are made for any drug or compound at present under clinical investigation.

Project manager: Lisa Langley
Designer: Joe Harvey and Taymoor Fouladi
Production: Marina Maher
Printed in Spain by Espace

Clinician's Manual on Ankylosing Spondylitis

Contents

Author biographies

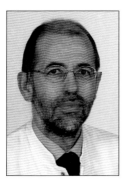

Joachim Sieper
Charité University Hospital
Berlin, Germany

Joachim Sieper, MD, is a Consultant and Head of Rheumatology at the Charité University Hospital, Campus Benjamin Franklin in Berlin, Germany. After receiving his medical degree in 1978 from Free University, in Berlin, Germany, he underwent his training in internal medicine in the Department of Cardiology at the Rudolf–Virchow clinic in Berlin, Germany. He continued his training in internal medicine and rheumatology at the University Hospital Benjamin Franklin, in Berlin, Germany. During this time he had a number of fellowships abroad including 8 weeks at The London Lupus Clinic, Hammersmith Hospital, in London, UK, led by Professor Graham Hughes. He also spent over a year at the Rheumatology Unit of Guy's Hospital, in London, UK, led by Professor G Panayi. In 1998 he became Professor of Medicine at Free University and that same year he was also appointed Deputy Head of the Department of Internal Medicine at the same institution. In 2000 he became Head of Rheumatology at Free University.

Professor Sieper is also a prolific researcher and writer. He has been an investigator since 1989, and a principal investigator since 1993 on several placebo-controlled randomised trials, which have been published internationally. He has authored and contributed to over 300 journal papers.

He is a member of numerous societies including the German Society of Rheumatology and the American College of Rheumatology.

He has also been the recipient of many awards and honours for excellence in rheumatology, including the Carol–Nachman award for rheumatology in 2000 and the European League Against Rheumatism (EULAR) award in 2003.

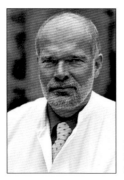

Jürgen Braun
Rheumatology Center Ruhrgebiet
Herne, Germany

Jürgen Braun, MD, is Medical Director of the Rheumatology Medical Centre, Ruhrgebiet in Herne, Germany, and is a lecturer at the Ruhr University in Bochum, Germany. He is also an honorary Professor in Rheumatology at the Charité Medical School in Berlin, Germany.

He received his doctor of medicine degree in 1987 at the Free University, Berlin, Germany, and went on to become certified as a specialist in rheumatology, internal medicine, laboratory medicine, physical therapy and sports medicine. In 2000, he became Professor of Rheumatology at the Free University, Berlin. The following year he became Medical Director of the Rheumatology Medical Centre, Ruhrgebiet in Herne, one of the major hospitals in Germany specialised in the management of patients with rheumatic diseases, a position he still holds.

Professor Braun has been an invited speaker at a number of universities and institutions including the National Institutes of Health, the American College of Rheumatology, the European League Against Rheumatism (EULAR), and the Asia Pacific League of Associations for Rheumatology. He has also been invited to speak about his research at the national meetings of the British, Irish, Indian, Scandinavian, Danish, Dutch, Belgian, Italian, Spanish, Greek, Turkish, Moroccan, Russian, Chinese, and German Society of Rheumatology. In 2004, he was appointed as the inaugural Robert Inman lecturer at the University of Toronto, Canada.

Professor Braun has been the recipient of several prestigious awards, including the Ankylosing Spondylitis Patients Association Award in 1996, the Tosse-Research Award in Pediatric Rheumatology in 1998, the Carol Nachman Research Award in 2000, and the EULAR prize in 2003.

As one of the leading specialists in the field of the spondyloarthritides, Professor Braun has published more than 300 papers on different aspects of this subject. He is a member of the Steering Committee of the Assessments in Ankylosing Spondylitis Working group and the Group for Research and Assessment of Psoriasis and Psoriatic Arthritis.

Acknowledgements

Our thanks go to our colleagues in the Assessment in SpondyloArthritis international Society (ASAS) for their permission to reproduce Figures 3.8, 4.3, 4.4, 4.5, 6.8 and 6.18 in this manual.

Abbreviations

AS	ankylosing spondylitis
ASAS	Assessment in SpondyloArthritis international Society
ASDAS	Ankylosing Spondylitis Disease Activity Score
ASSERT	Ankylosing Spondylitis Study for the Evaluation of Recombinant infliximab Therapy study
BASDAI	Bath Ankylosing Spondylitis Disease Activity Index
BASMI	Bath Ankylosing Spondylitis Metrology Index
BASFI	Bath Ankylosing Spondylitis Functional Index
COX-2	cyclooxygenase 2
CRP	C-reactive protein
CT	computed tomography
CV	cardiovascular
DISH	diffuse idiopathic skeletal hyperostosis
DMARD	disease-modifying anti-rheumatic drug
ESR	erythrocyte sedimentation rate
ESSG	European Spondylarthropathy Study Group
EULAR	European League Against Rheumatism
GI	gastrointestinal
HLA	human leukocyte antigen
IBD	inflammatory bowel disease
IBP	inflammatory back pain
IL	interleukin
JIA	juvenile idiopathic arthritis
LR	likelihood ratio
MASES	Maastricht Ankylosing Spondylitis Enthesitis Score
MRI	magnetic resonance imaging
NRS	numerical rating scale
NSAID	nonsteroidal anti-inflammatory drug
PsA	psoriatic arthritis
SI	sacroiliac
SpA	spondyloarthritis
STIR	short tau inversion recovery
TB	tuberculosis
Th-17	T-helper cell 17
TNF	tumour necrosis factor
TNF-α	tumour necrosis factor alpha
VAS	visual analogue scale

Chapter 1

Introduction

Only slightly more common in men than in women, ankylosing spondylitis (AS) is a chronic inflammatory disease which, probably as a result of an autoimmune response, causes inflammation in the sacroiliac joints, vertebrae and adjacent joints. Patients also frequently have inflammation of an enthesis (insertion of a tendon or ligament into the bone), the peripheral joints and the eye; the lungs, heart valves and kidneys are only rarely affected. The onset of symptoms – notably back pain and stiffness – is normally already noticeable in adolescence or early adulthood. Eventually, AS can cause the vertebrae to fuse together, with obvious adverse impact on patient mobility and function. To date, the disease has no cure, but drug and physical therapy can improve pain, inflammation and other symptoms considerably; indeed, even remission is now a realistic goal. A major breakthrough in the treatment of this disease was the demonstration of the high efficacy of the tumour necrosis factor (TNF)-blocking agents [1].

The diagnosis of AS is often delayed as symptoms can be confused with other more common, but normally less serious, disorders because chronic low back pain is such a common complaint. Furthermore, typical radiological changes of the sacroiliac joint become visible only after some time, often years, of ongoing inflammation. Therefore, it is proposed that the term 'axial spondyloarthritis' be used, which covers both patients with ankylosing spondylitis and those with non-radiographic sacroiliitis. Early accurate diagnosis and intervention can, however, minimize or even prevent years of pain and disability. In the face of these challenges, the *Clinician's Manual on Ankylosing Spondylitis* provides a concise, clinically focused overview of the manifestations, diagnosis and management of this potentially debilitating condition.

A historical perspective

Studies of Egyptian mummies indicate that the disease now known as AS has afflicted humankind since antiquity. The first historical description of

AS appeared in the literature in 1559, when Realdo Colombo provided an anatomical description of two skeletons with abnormalities typical of AS. More than 100 years later, the Irish doctor Bernard Connor described a bony fusion of spine and sacroiliac joints of a human skeleton. Despite several descriptions of conditions resembling AS later on, the reports of Bechterew in Russia (1893), Strümpell in Germany (1897) and Marie in France (1898) are often cited as the first descriptions of AS. Around 1900 the terms 'Bechterew's disease', used preferentially in German-speaking countries and Russia, and 'ankylosing spondylitis' were introduced.

At this time a diagnosis could be made only when an AS patient had already developed the typical posture (see Figure 1.1a) that results from an advanced ankylosis of the spine or *post mortem*. It was not until the 1930s that roentgenology was applied to AS, and it became evident from these studies that, in about 95% of cases, the sacroiliac joint is affected in AS (Figure 1.1b). These findings are the basis for the prominent role of radiographic sacroiliitis in the currently used diagnostic and classification criteria for AS, such as the 1984 modified New York criteria [2]. However, there was already some evidence, both clinically and from scintigraphy, that patients may have symptoms caused by inflammation many years before structural damage becomes visible on radiographs. The presence of an inflammatory non(pre)-radiographic stage early in the course of the disease became much clearer when magnetic resonance imaging (MRI) was used in AS in the 1990s (Figure 1.1c) [3]. Consequently, acute inflammatory sacroiliitis shown by MRI has become part of the new classification criteria for axial spondyloarthritis.

Starting in the 1920s radiation treatment was used for AS patients to treat spinal pain and had good results such as improvement of the symptoms. However, this therapy was abandoned because of the serious long-term side effects of such treatment, such as leukaemia and other malignancies. Although treatment with salicylates has been used for the treatment of inflammatory rheumatic diseases since about 1900, this drug was not effective in AS. Phenylbutazone was introduced into clinical practice in 1949 and became the first drug to which the term 'non-steroidal anti-inflammatory drug' (NSAID) was applied. It has been highly effective for the treatment of AS with control of pain and inflammation. However, its use has been restricted to only short-term treatment of AS because of potentially serious side effects, notably aplastic anaemia and hepatic injury. Subsequently, since around 1965 a second generation of NSAIDs, led by indometacin, has been successfully used in the treatment of AS up to the present. Finally, the high efficacy of TNF-blocker treatment was demonstrated in AS patients in the first years of the new century.

Historical aspects of AS

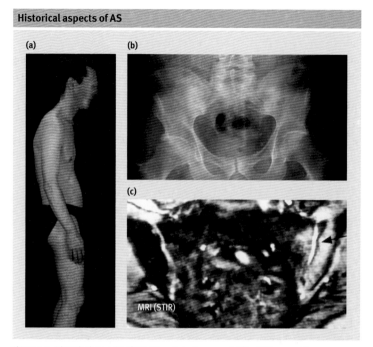

Figure 1.1. Historical aspects of AS. AS, ankylosing spondylitis; MRI, magnetic resonance imaging; STIR, short tau inversion recovery. **(a)** in the 1900s a diagnosis could only be made when the patient exhibited the typical posture associated with AS; **(b)** a radiograph showing bilateral sacroilitis - roentgenology began to be applied to AS in the 1930s; **(c)** a magnetic resonance image showing a patient with acute sacroiliitis – the use of MRI in the early 1990s helped to identify the presence of an inflammatory non-radiographic stage early in the course of AS.

Chapter 2

Overview of ankylosing spondylitis

The concept and classification of spondyloarthritis

The term 'spondyloarthritis' (SpA) comprises AS, reactive arthritis, arthritis/spondylitis associated with psoriasis, and arthritis/spondylitis associated with inflammatory bowel disease (IBD). There is considerable overlap between the single subsets (Figure 2.1). The main link between each is the association with the human leukocyte antigen (HLA)-B27, the same pattern of peripheral joint involvement with an asymmetrical, often pauciarticular, arthritis, predominantly of the lower limbs, and the possible occurrence of sacroiliitis, spondylitis, enthesitis, dactylitis and uveitis. All SpA subsets can evolve into AS, especially in those patients who are positive for HLA-B27. The SpA subsets can also be split into patients with predominantly axial and predominantly peripheral SpA (Figure 2.2), with an overlap between the two parts in about 20–40% of cases. Through use of such a classification the presence or absence of evidence for a preceding gastrointestinal or urogenital infection, psoriasis or IBD is recorded but does not result in a different classification. The term 'predominant axial SpA' covers patients with classic AS and those with non-radiographic axial SpA [4]. The latter group of patients would not have radiographic sacroiliitis according to the modified New York criteria, but would normally have evidence of active inflammation as shown by magnetic resonance imaging (MRI) or other means (discussed in more detail in Chapter 5).

The concept of 'seronegative spondarthritides', now known as 'spondyloarthritides', was first introduced in 1974 by Moll and Wright from Leeds. 'Seronegative' stands here for rheumatoid factor negative. Subsequently, both the European Spondyloarthropathy Study Group (ESSG) classification criteria and the Amor criteria (from the French rheumatologist Bernard Amor) tried to define the whole spectrum of SpA [5, 6]. It was thanks to the ESSG criteria that in 1991 the SpA group was first split into predominantly axial and peripheral subsets. Figure 2.3 shows the current ESSG classification criteria for spondyloarthritis. Most recently the Assessment in SpondyloArthritis international Society (ASAS) has proposed new classification criteria on axial spondyloarthritis, a term that is used throughout this book [7].

Epidemiology of ankylosing spondylitis

AS is a disease that starts normally in the third decade of life, with about 80% of patients developing the first symptoms before the age of 30 and less than 5% of patients being older than 45 at the start of the disease. Up to 20% of patients are even younger than 20 years when they experience their first symptoms (Figure 2.4) [8]. Patients who are positive for HLA-B27 are about 10 years younger than HLA-B27-negative patients when the disease starts [9].

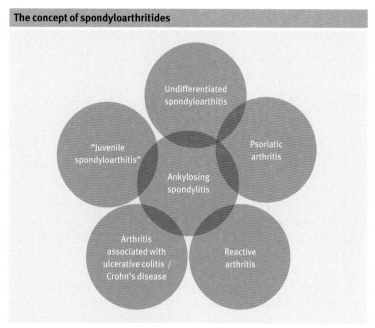

The concept of spondyloarthritides

Undifferentiated spondyloarthitis

"Juvenile spondyloarthitis"

Psoriatic arthritis

Ankylosing spondylitis

Arthritis associated with ulcerative colitis / Crohn's disease

Reactive arthritis

Figure 2.1 The concept of spondyloarthritides.

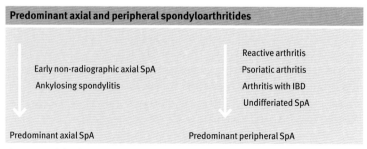

Predominant axial and peripheral spondyloarthritides

Early non-radiographic axial SpA

Ankylosing spondylitis

Reactive arthritis

Psoriatic arthritis

Arthritis with IBD

Undifferiated SpA

Predominant axial SpA

Predominant peripheral SpA

Figure 2.2 Axial and peripheral spondyloarthritides. IBD, inflammatory bowel disease; SpA, spondyloarthritis. Data from Rudwaleit et al. [4].

ESSG classification criteria for spondyloarthropathy

Inflammatory back pain	or	Synovitis
		• asymmetrical or
		• predominantly in the lower limbs

plus one of the following:

• alternating buttock pain

• sacroiliitis

• heel pain (enthesitis)

• positive family history

• psoriasis

• Crohn's disease, ulcerative colitis

• urethritis / acute diarrhea in the preceding 4 weeks

Figure 2.3 ESSG classification criteria for spondyloarthropathy. ESSG, European Spondyloarthropathy Study Group. Data from Dougados et al. [5].

Age at first symptoms and at first diagnosis in patients with AS

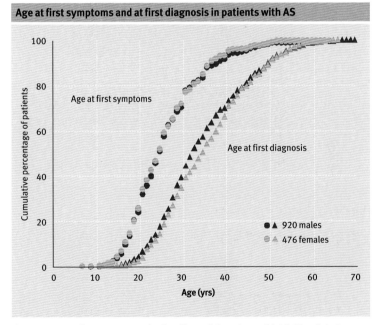

Figure 2.4 Age at first symptoms and at first diagnosis in patients with AS. AS, ankylosing spondylitis. Reproduced with permission from Feldtkeller et al [8].

Men are slightly more affected than are women, with a ratio of about 2:1. However, women develop chronic radiographic changes of the sacroiliac joints and the spine later than men, a possible explanation for the frequent under-diagnosis of AS in women in the past, resulting in a much higher male:female ratio than currently accepted [9].

There is a clear correlation between the prevalence of HLA-B27 and the prevalence of AS in a given population: the higher the HLA-B27 prevalence the higher the AS prevalence. HLA-B27 is present throughout the world with a wide ethnic and geographical variation. It is most prevalent in northern countries and some tribes (Figure 2.5). Overall, estimations about the prevalence of AS

Prevalence of AS

Country	AS prevalence	HLA-B27 prevalence
US*	1.0–1.5%	8%
The Netherlands†	0.1%	8%
Germany‡	0.55%	9%
Norway§	1.1–1.4%	14%
Haida Indians¶	6.1%	50%

Figure 2.5 Prevalence of AS. AS, ankylosing spondylitis; HLA, human leukocyte antigen. *Data from Calin et al. [10]; †Data from van der Linden et al. [11]; ‡Data from Braun et al. [12]; §Data from Gran et al. [13]; ¶Data from Gofton et al. [14].

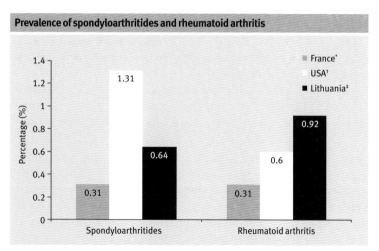

Figure 2.6 Prevalence of spondyloarthritides and rheumatoid arthritis.
*Data from Saraux et al. [15] and Guillemin et al. [16]; †Data from Adomaviciute et al. [17]; ‡Helmick et al. [18].

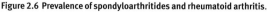

are between 0.1% and 1.4%, with most of these data coming from Europe. In western and mid-Europe a prevalence of 0.3–0.5% for AS and of 1–2% for the whole SpA group is likely. Recent studies from France, the USA and Lithuania indicate that SpA is at least as common as rheumatoid arthritis (Figure 2.6), which makes AS and SpA one of the most important chronic inflammatory rheumatic diseases [15–19].

HLA-B27 is positive in 90–95% of AS patients and in about 80–90% of patients with non-radiographic axial SpA. This percentage goes down to about 60% in AS patients who also have psoriasis or IBD. In predominant peripheral SpA, less than 50% of patients are positive for HLA-B27.

Aetiopathogenesis of ankylosing spondylitis

A major breakthrough in the research on the pathogenesis of AS and related SpA was the reported strong association of the disease with HLA-B27 in 1973 [20]. However, intensive research over more than three decades has not clarified the functional role of the HLA-B27 molecule in the pathogenic process. In the centre of the discussion about pathogenesis of SpA is the interaction between bacteria and HLA-B27, as a result of known triggering bacteria in reactive arthritis (after preceding bacterial infections of the urogenital or gastrointestinal tract) and the association with IBD; in the latter the immune system can interact with local gut bacteria because of a damaged mucosa [21]. Between 10% and 50% of HLA-B27-positive patients with reactive arthritis or IBD develop AS over the years, supporting a central role for such an interaction between bacteria and HLA-B27 in its pathogenesis. Although in most AS patients no bacterial exposure can be detected, subclinical bacterial infection or gut inflammation would be a possibility in these patients.

Many recent MRI studies and older pathological investigations suggest that the primary target of the immune response is at the cartilage/bone interface, including the insertion of tendon and ligaments at the bone (enthesis) [22]. Such an immunopathology would most probably differ from rheumatoid arthritis, in which inflammation occurs primarily in the synovium. We have recently provided further evidence for this hypothesis, showing that the presence of mononuclear cell infiltrates and osteoclasts depends on the presence of cartilage on the joint surface in AS patients (Figure 2.7) [23]. However, there is currently no evidence that bacteria or bacterial antigens persist in the cartilage or close to the cartilage of spine and joints. Thus, there have been speculations that bacteria might trigger an autoimmune response against cartilage-derived antigens such as proteoglycan or collagen, possibly mediated somehow through HLA-B27, although this hypothesis has not yet been proved. A third and necessary triggering component could be microtrauma(s) of cartilage/ bone because weight-bearing parts of the skeleton are almost exclusively affected in AS.

In addition to inflammation, AS is also characterized by new bone formation, with the possible consequence of bone fusion, most frequently found in the axial skeleton in the form of syndesmophytes. For a long time there has been a question over how inflammation and new bone formation are coupled in AS, whether AS is a disease of excessive new bone formation or whether this is only part of a physiological repair mechanism. Figure 2.8 shows a likely sequence of events: first inflammation causes an osteitis, followed by erosive structural damage of bone and cartilage, which are filled up with (fibrous) repair tissue, with a final step in which this repair tissue is subsequently ossified. If this is true, new bone formation would not occur without previous erosive damage from inflammation [24–26]. Further research is necessary to clarify the pathogenesis of AS and the characteristic interaction between inflammation and new bone formation.

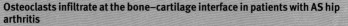

Osteoclasts infiltrate at the bone–cartilage interface in patients with AS hip arthritis

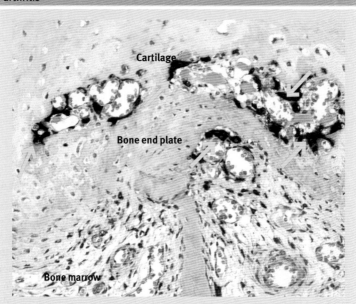

Figure 2.7 Osteoclasts infiltrate at the bone–cartilage interface in patients with AS hip arthritis. AS, ankylosing spondylitis. Osteoclasts are shown in red (arrows). From Appel et al. [25].

Proposed sequence of structural damage in AS

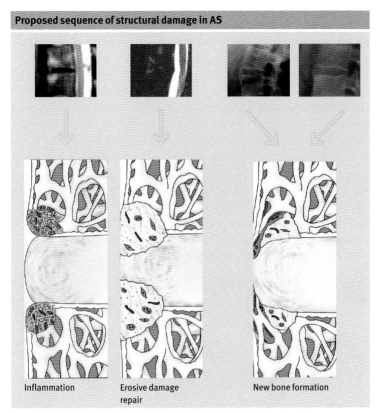

| Inflammation | Erosive damage repair | | New bone formation |

Figure 2.8 **Proposed sequence of structural damage in AS**. From Appel et al. [25].

Genetics of ankylosing spondylitis

Susceptibility to AS has been estimated to be genetically determined in more than 90% of cases, and it has been suggested that, as a result, there might not be a single factor, such as one bacterium, but ubiquitous environmental factors, (eg, many different bacteria) [27]. By far the strongest genetic association is with HLA-B27, and more than 30 HLA-B27 subtypes have been described to date. Some of them, such as HLA-B*2706 and HLA-B*2709, are either not associated, or less associated, with the disease, suggesting that minor molecular differences between the molecules might be the key to a better understanding of the pathogenesis. Although differentiation of HLA-B27 subtypes is of research interest, it has no clinical value and should therefore not be applied in daily clinical practice.

Most recently two new genetic loci have been shown to be associated with AS: interleukin receptor IL-23R, which is involved in the Th-17 (T-helper cell 17) pathway of chronic immune responses, and ARTS-1 (endoplasmic reticulum aminopeptidase 1), an enzyme that is relevant for the processing of peptides in the cytoplasm [28]. The relative contribution of these genes to the susceptibility to AS can be compared by using the population-attributable risk fraction statistic, which is 90% for HLA-B27, 26% for ARTS-1 and 9% for IL-23 [28]. Other factors such as HLA-B60, IL-1A and *CYP2D6* (cytochrome P450 2D6) have been described as affecting the risk of developing AS, although this is not completely clear.

Only about 5% of HLA-B27-positive individuals develop AS. The average risk of developing AS in a first-degree relative (children or sibling) of an AS patient is about 8%, although only 1% or less of second- and third-degree relatives are affected. The risk can be better estimated when the HLA-B27 status is known: about 12% in HLA-B27-positive first-degree relatives, but less than 1% in HLA-B27-negative relatives (Figure 2.9) [29].

Risk of developing AS in a first-degree relative	
HLA-B27 status	**Risk (%)**
Negative	<1
Positive	12
Unknown	8

Figure 2.9 Risk of developing AS in a first-degree relative. AS, ankylosing spondylitis; HLA, human leukocyte antigen. Data from Brown et al. [29].

Chapter 3

Clinical manifestations of ankylosing spondylitis

Inflammatory back pain

The main clinical symptoms in AS are pain and stiffness of the back, predominantly of the lower back and the pelvis, but any part of the spine can be involved. Typical for AS/spondyloarthritis (SpA) is inflammatory back pain (IBP) which is defined clinically and not by laboratory tests such as C-reactive protein (CRP) or erythrocyte sedimentation rate (ESR). Patients complain about morning stiffness of the back, with improvement on exercise but not by rest. In addition, or alternatively, they report awakening at night, mostly in the second half of the night, because of back pain which improves on getting up and moving around (Figure 3.1). Furthermore, back pain should be chronic (>3 months duration) not acute, and it should occur for the first time before the age of 45 years, because the disease starts at a young age; this also helps to differentiate it from degenerative spine disease, the prevalence of which increases with age. Most patients report a mixture of pain and stiffness in the spine, although either can be the main or only symptom.

Various sets of criteria for IBP have been proposed and applied combining the parameters mentioned above and shown in Figure 3.2 [30–32]. They also performed well when investigated in studies, although all have a limited sensitivity and specificity. A sensitivity of no more than 80% implies that 20% of AS patients do not complain about characteristic IBP,

Characteristics of inflammatory back pain
• Morning stiffness of the back >30 min
• Awakening in the second half of the night because of back pain
• Improvement of pain and stiffness by exercise but not by rest
• Chronic back pain (>3 months duration) starting at an age <45 years

Figure 3.1 Characteristics of inflammatory back pain.

and a specificity no higher than 80% means that 20% of control patients (eg patients with mechanically induced low back pain) complain about, for example, morning stiffness with improvement through exercise [33]. Nevertheless, IBP is an important clinical criterion in AS/SpA.

Inflammatory back pain defined according to various criteria		
Calin et al.[1]	Rudwaleit et al.[2]	IBP experts (ASAS)[3]
• age at onset <40 yrs	• morning stiffness >30 min	• age at onset <40 yrs
• duration of back pain >3 months	• improvement with exercise, not with rest	• insidious onset
		• improvement with exercise
• insidious onset	• awakening at 2nd half of the night because of pain	• no improvement with rest
• morning stiffness		• pain at night (with improvement upon getting up)
• improvement with exercise	• alternating buttock pain	
IBP if 4 / 5 are present.	IBP if 2 / 4 are present.	IBP if 4 / 5 are present.

Figure 3.2 Inflammatory back pain defined according to various criteria.
ASAS, Assessment in SpondyloArthritis international Society; IBP, inflammatory back pain.
[1]Data from Calin et al. [30]; [2]Data from Rudwaleit et al. [32]; [3]Data from Sieper et al. [31].

Restriction of spinal mobility

Further in the course of the disease, syndesmophytes and ossification of the facet joints can develop, resulting in restriction of spinal mobility. The long-term outcome is strongly determined by restriction of spinal mobility. However, not all AS patients have syndesmophytes. In AS patients with a disease (symptom) duration of less than 10 years syndesmophytes are detectable in only about 25%, and in patients with a mean disease duration of more than 20 years syndesmophytes are visible on radiographs in about 60% [9, 34]. A recent study showed that both disease activity and radiographic damage of the spine determine function independently, with disease activity being more relevant earlier in the course of the disease [35]. Measurement and documentation of spinal mobility, as shown in Figures 3.3–3.7, are recommended in the follow-up of AS patients.

In addition to restriction of spinal mobility patients can develop flexion contractures of hip and knee joints, which together result in a characteristic posture for advanced disease in AS patients (see Figure 1.1a).

Modified Schober test to asess motion of the lumbar spine

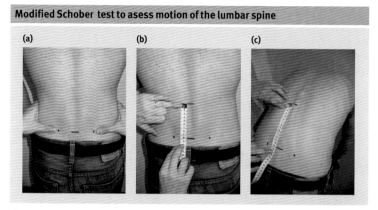

Figure 3.3 **Modified Schober test to assess motion of the lumbar spine**. **(a)** the patient stands erect and the clinician marks an imaginary line connecting both posterior superior iliac spines (close to the dimples of Venus); **(b)** another mark is placed 10 cm above; **(c)** the patient bends forward maximally, and the difference is measured. The best of two attempts is recorded and the increase in centimetres is recorded to the nearest 0.1cm.

Measuring lateral spinal flexion

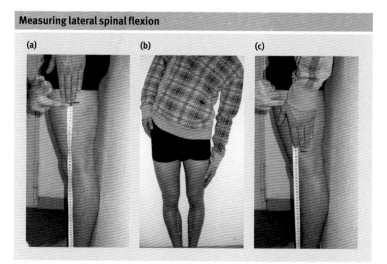

Figure 3.4 **Measuring lateral spinal flexion**. **(a)** the patient rests their heels and back against the wall, with no flexion in the knees and without bending forward and the clinician marks the thigh; **(b)** the patient bends sideways without bending their knees or lifting their heels; **(c)** the clinician places a second mark and records the difference.

Measuring cervical and thoracic spine extension: occiput-to-wall and tragus-to-wall distance

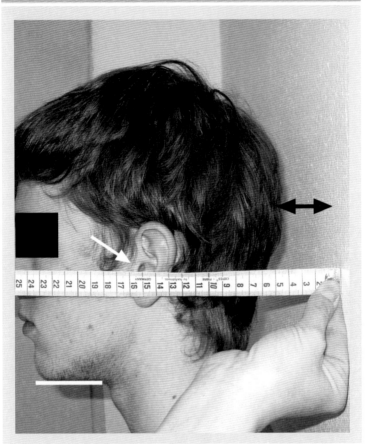

Figure 3.5 Measuring cervical and thoracic spine extension: occiput-to-wall and tragus-to-wall distance. The heels and back rest against the wall, with the chin at usual carrying level. The patient tries to touch the head against the wall. The best of two tries is recorded in centimetres (eg, 10.2cm). The occiput-to-wall (black arrow) or tragus-to-wall (white arrow) distance can be measured.

Measuring cervical rotation to assess neck mobility in patients with AS

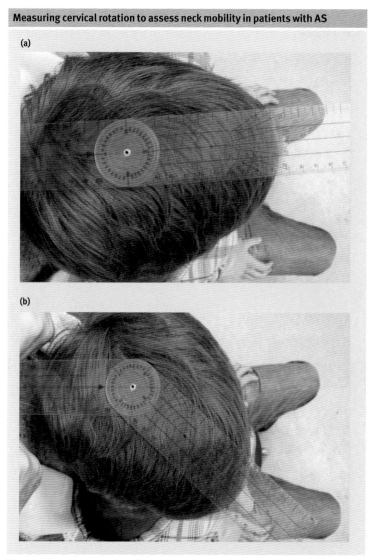

Figure 3.6 Measuring cervical rotation to assess neck mobility in patients with AS.
AS, ankylosing spondylitis. **(a)** the patient sits straight on a chair, chin level, hands on the knees. The assessor places a goniometer at the top of the head in line with the nose; **(b)** the assessor asks the patient to rotate the neck maximally to the left, follows with the goniometer, and records the angle between the sagital plane and the new plane after rotation. A second reading is taken and the best of the two is recorded for the left side. The procedure is repeated for the right side. The mean of left and right is recorded in degrees (0–90°) (normal >70°).

Chest expansion

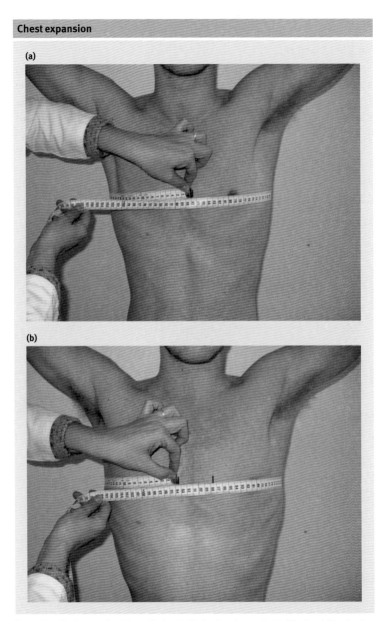

Figure 3.7 Chest expansion. The patient rests his/her hands on or behind the head. The chest is measured at the fourth intercostal level anteriorly. **(a)** the maximal inspiration is recorded; **(b)** the maximal expiration is recorded. The difference is recorded in centimetres (eg, 4.3cm) and the best of two tries is noted.

Extraspinal rheumatic manifestations
Peripheral arthritis

Peripheral arthritis occurs frequently, but often transiently, in AS and presents typically as an asymmetrical arthritis and/or as an arthritis predominantly of the lower limbs (Figure 3.8). In a cohort of AS patients with a mean symptom duration of 18 years, 58% of patients reported a peripheral arthritis [36]. This figure was slightly lower in an AS cohort with a symptom duration of less than 10 years, with 37.4% of patients reporting arthritis, but only 14.4% of patients reporting it at the time of presentation [9]. The pattern of peripheral joint involvement in one study was oligoarthritis (fewer than five joints) in 55%, monoarthritis in 24% and polyarthritis in 21% [36].

Acute gonarthritis in a patient with peripheral spondyloarthritis

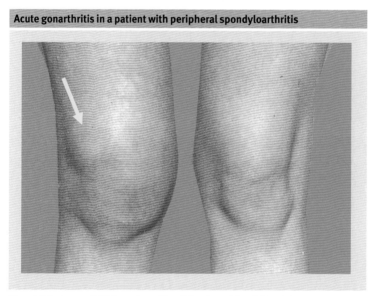

Figure 3.8 **Acute gonarthritis in a patient with peripheral spondyloarthritis.** The knee on the left shows a patient with peripheral spondyloarthritis (arrow) while the knee on the right is normal. Figure provided courtesy of ASAS.

Enthesitis

Enthesitis (inflammation at the insertion of tendons, ligaments or capsules into bone) is also a frequent manifestation in AS and occurred in 50% of a cohort with long-standing AS and in 39.4% of a cohort with shorter disease duration [9, 36]. The percentage of patients with enthesitis at presentation was 21% in the latter cohort. The lower limbs are most frequently affected, especially at the insertion of Achilles' tendon and/or the plantar fascia at the calcaneus (Figure 3.9). However, inflammation is possible at any enthesial site.

Enthesitis in the right heel of a patient

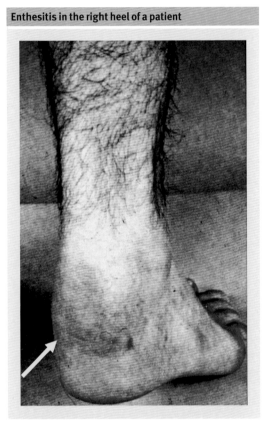

Figure 3.9 Enthesitis in the right heel of a patient.
Insertion of Achilles tendon at calcaneus.

Enthesitis in peripheral joints

The sites affected by inflammation in peripheral joints can be both the synovium and the insertion of tendons/ligaments at bone. Figure 3.10 shows a good example of both subchondral bone marrow oedema and effusion in an SpA patient with gonarthritis, compared with a patient with rheumatoid arthritis with no bone marrow oedema. This implies that a peripheral joint in SpA might not be swollen, only painful (especially pain on local pressure and, if accessible, on movement).

Hip and shoulder joints

Involvement of the hip and shoulder joints is frequent, but often regarded as part of the axial skeleton manifestation and not as peripheral arthritis. Hip involvement was reported in 27% of AS patients with longstanding disease [36] and it can be expected that about 5% of AS patients have to undergo hip joint replacement in the course of their disease as a result of arthritis of the hip and

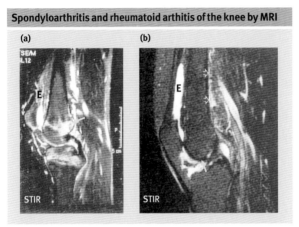
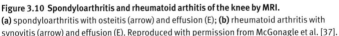

Figure 3.10 Spondyloarthritis and rheumatoid arthitis of the knee by MRI.
(a) spondyloarthritis with osteitis (arrow) and effusion (E); **(b)** rheumatoid arthritis with synovitis (arrow) and effusion (E). Reproduced with permission from McGonagle et al. [37].

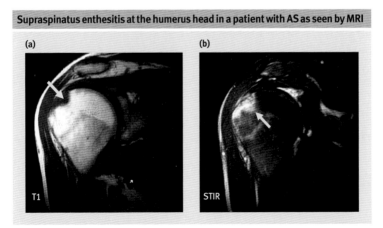

Figure 3.11 Supraspinatus enthesitis at the humerus head in a patient with AS as seen by MRI.
AS, ankylosing spondylitis; MRI, magnetic resonance image; STIR, short tau inversion recovery.
(a) bone marrow oedema: hypointense on T1; **(b)** bone marrow oedema: hyperintense on STIR.
Reproduced with permission from Lambert et al. [38].

secondary osteoarthritis. In one study, shoulder pain was reported in 3.5% and shoulder involvement by clinical evaluation in 25% [38]. Rotator cuff tendonitis and enthesitis at the insertion of the supraspinatus tendon at the greater tuberosity of the humerus (Figure 3.11) and enthesitis at the acromial origin of the deltoid muscle were the most frequently found abnormalities, when patients were examined by MRI [38]. Bone marrow oedema was the most characteristic finding while effusion was rare.

Dactylitis

Dactylitis is a swelling of a finger or toe as a consequence of a tendovaginitis (Figure 3.12). It is typical for the whole group of SpA but it is more rare in AS (dactylitis in 6.3% in one study [36]) than it is in psoriatic arthritis.

Dactylitis in a patient with psoriasis

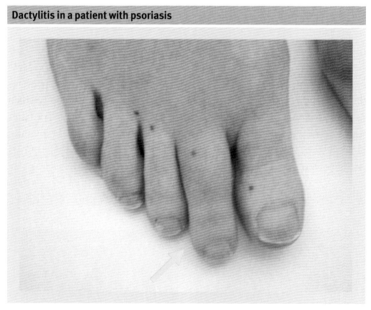

Figure 3.12 **Dactylitis in a patient with psoriasis**. Swelling of the second toe in a patient with psoriasis.

Extraarticular locations

Uveitis anterior is the most frequent extraarticular location in AS, which occurs in about 30% of AS patients. This percentage was lower (21%) in AS patients with a symptom duration of less than 10 years. The percentage of patients with uveitis at presentation is rather small (1.7% in one study) [9].

The typical clinical picture of uveitis is predominantly anterior, unilateral, sudden in onset, limited in duration, and often alternating from one eye to the other (Figure 3.13) [39].

The presence or history of psoriasis is reported in about 10% of AS patients and the presence or history of inflammatory bowel disease is reported in 3–10%, with an increasing frequency found over time.

Clinical characteristics of uveitis anterior in AS
• Acute (self-limiting)
• Unilateral
• Sudden in onset (painful and red eye)
• Alternating from one eye to the other

Figure 3.13 Clinical characteristics of uveitis anterior in AS. AS, ankylosing spondylitis.

Juvenile-onset spondyloarthritis

In up to 20% of AS patients the disease starts before the age of 20 years and a diagnosis of juvenile-onset SpA can be made in up to 50% of patients presenting with juvenile idiopathic arthritis (JIA). Paediatricians prefer the term 'enthesitis-related arthritis' rather than juvenile-onset SpA, which describes a similar, although not identical, subset of patients [40]. The latter term makes it clearer that juvenile-onset SpA and adult SpA are a continuum of the same disease. The clinical picture is dominated by peripheral arthritis and enthesitis of the lower limbs. Spondylitis, sacroiliitis and extraarticular problems are not frequent in childhood but evolve over time [41]. About 60–80% of HLA-B27-positive juvenile SpA patients develop AS and other chronic spondyloarthritides 10 years after onset.

Chapter 4

Diagnosis of ankylosing spondylitis

The modified New York criteria

According to the modified New York criteria, which are still widely used, the hallmark for the diagnosis of AS has been the detection of sacroiliitis by radiographs (Figure 4.1) [2]. Sacroiliitis is graded using a scoring system as shown in Figure 4.2. A diagnosis of AS can be made if sacroiliitis grade 2 bilaterally or grade 3 or higher unilaterally is present together with one clinical criterion, such as the presence of the clinical symptom inflammatory back pain or restriction of spinal mobility. As spinal involvement with the development of syndesmophytes normally occurs later in the course of the disease and as the spine is rarely affected without the sacroiliac (SI) joint, radiographic changes of the spine are not part of these diagnostic criteria. Examples of normal and abnormal sacroiliac joints are shown in Figures 4.3–4.5.

Modified New York criteria for AS
1. Clinical criteria
• Low back pain and stiffness >3 months which improves with exercise, but is not relieved by rest
• Limitation of motion of the lumbar spine in both the sagittal and frontal planes
• Limitation of chest expansion relative to normal values correlated for age and sex
2. Radiological criterion
Sacroiliitis grade ≥2 bilaterally or grade 3–4 unilaterally
Definite AS if the radiological criterion is associated with at least 1 clinical criterion.

Figure 4.1 Modified New York criteria for AS. AS, ankylosing spondylitis.
Data from van der Linden et al. [11].

Grading of radiographic sacroiliitis

Grade 0	Normal
Grade 1	Suspicious changes
Grade 2	Minimal abnormality – small localised areas with erosion or sclerosis, without alteration in the joint width
Grade 3	Unequivocal abnormality – moderate or advanced sacroiliitis with one or more of: erosions, evidence of sclerosis, widening, narrowing, or partial ankylosis.
Grade 4	Severe abnormality – total ankylosis

Figure 4.2 Grading of radiographic sacroiliitis. Data from Bennett et al. [42].

Sacroilitis grade 0 normal

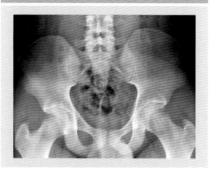

Figure 4.3 Sacroiliitis grade 0 normal. Figure provided courtesy of ASAS.

Sacroiliitis grade 1 and 2

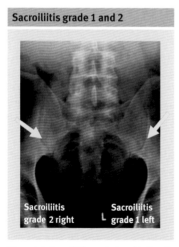

Sacroiliitis grade 2 right

Sacroiliitis grade 1 left

Figure 4.4 Sacroiliitis grade 1 and 2. A patient with grade 1 sacroiliitis on the left and grade 2 sacroiliitis on the right. Figure provided courtesy of ASAS.

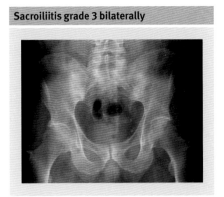

Sacroiliitis grade 3 bilaterally

Figure 4.5 Sacroiliitis grade 3 bilaterally. Figure provided courtesy of ASAS.

Delay between onset of symptoms and diagnosis

There is currently an unacceptably long delay between the first occurrence of AS symptoms and a diagnosis of AS being made 5–10 years afterwards (see Figure 2.4) [8]. This results in young patients with chronic back pain frequently consulting many different doctors (because patients are not getting a diagnosis), having redundant and potentially expensive diagnostic procedures and treatments and, most importantly, having a major delay in starting effective therapy.

There are two major reasons for such a delay: the first is that there is certainly a low awareness of AS among non-rheumatologists and it can also be seen as a major challenge for any doctor in primary care to think of and identify patients with inflammatory spine disease among the large group of patients with chronic back pain, most often of other origin. To change this, the awareness of the disease among non-specialists has to be increased and effective programmes for screening of patients with chronic back pain for inflammatory spinal disease have to be incorporated into primary care. Possible solutions and first results are presented later in the chapter (see 'Screening for axial SpA' on page 35).

Second, radiographic sacroiliitis is usually a requirement for making a diagnosis of AS according to the modified New York criteria, as discussed earlier. However, radiographic changes indicate chronic changes and damage of the bone, and are the consequence of inflammation and not active inflammation itself. AS is a slowly progressive disease in terms of radiographic changes, and definite sacroiliitis on plain radiographs appears relatively late, often following several years of continuous or relapsing inflammation [4].

Figure 4.6 shows an estimated correlation between length of symptoms and the development of radiographic changes. Only a small proportion of patients will already have radiographic sacroiliitis at their first visit to the doctor, probably as a result of ongoing subclinical inflammation (A in Figure 4.6). After about 5 years roughly half the patients will already have radiographic sacroiliitis, but the other half will not (B in Figure 4.6). A smaller proportion of patients develop radiographic changes later (C in Figure 4.6) or never (D in Figure 4.6). Thus, for early diagnosis radiographic changes of the SI joints have a very limited role.

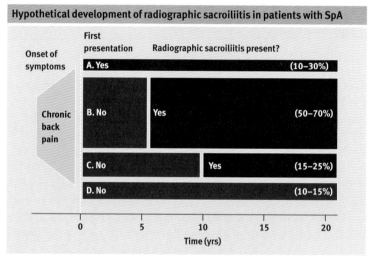

Figure 4.6 Hypothetical development of radiographic sacroiliitis in patients with SpA.
SpA, spondyloarthritis. Reproduced with permission from Rudwaleit et al. [4].

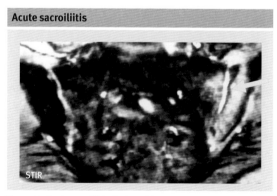

Figure 4.7 Acute sacroiliitis. Patient with acute sacroilitis on the left (arrow).

In early disease with no definite radiographic changes, active inflammation of SI joints can normally be visualised using magnetic resonance imaging (MRI) technology. The hallmark of a 'positive MRI' is the presence of subchondral bone marrow oedema, as shown in Figure 4.7 and discussed in more detail in Chapter 5 [43]. Clinical experience but also limited data suggest that a good proportion of patients with inflammation of the SI joints on MRI, but normal or suspicious radiographs, will develop radiographic sacroiliitis later on, which therefore evolves to AS [44]. Therefore, we have proposed that all patients with spondyloarthritis (SpA) with predominant axial involvement, irrespective of the presence or absence of radiographic changes, should be considered as belonging to one disease continuum (Figure 4.8) [4]. Furthermore, we have proposed the use of the term 'pre-radiographic' or 'non-radiographic axial SpA' for the group of patients with early axial SpA. Such a term is also preferable compared with 'undifferentiated (axial) SpA' because this subgroup is now well defined and can be diagnosed with no problems.

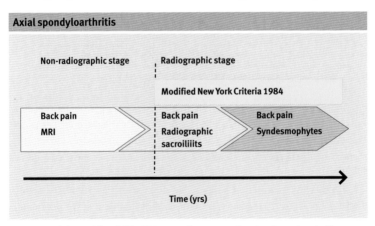

Figure 4.8 Axial spondyloarthritis. MRI, magnetic resonance imaging. Reproduced with permission from Rudwaleit et al. [4].

Following this reasoning, new criteria for the classification of axial SpA have been developed and are shown in Figures 4.9 and 4.10 [7]. Sacroiliitis, as seen on imaging, is still a crucial part of these criteria, but it can be detected by either radiographs (indicating chronic damage) or MRI (which is new!), showing active inflammation of the SI joint. Thus, radiographic sacroiliitis, as defined by the modified New York criteria, is part of, but not essential to, the classification. In addition to identifying sacroiliitis by imaging, one of the typical features of SpA has to be present (Figure 4.9). Restriction of spinal mobility, which is one of the clinical criteria for the modified New York criteria, is no longer part of the new criteria. Patients can also be classified as axial SpA in the absence of imaging results if three clinical parameters, including HLA-B27 positivity, are present.

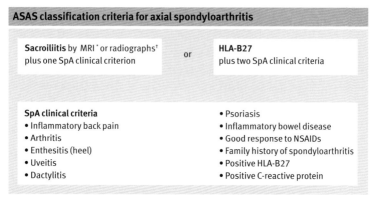

ASAS classification criteria for axial spondyloarthritis

Sacroiliitis by MRI* or radiographs† plus one SpA clinical criterion	or	HLA-B27 plus two SpA clinical criteria

SpA clinical criteria
- Inflammatory back pain
- Arthritis
- Enthesitis (heel)
- Uveitis
- Dactylitis

- Psoriasis
- Inflammatory bowel disease
- Good response to NSAIDs
- Family history of spondyloarthritis
- Positive HLA-B27
- Positive C-reactive protein

Figure 4.9 ASAS classification criteria for axial spondyloarthritis. ASAS, Assessment in SpondyloArthritis international Society; HLA, human leukocyte antigen; MRI, magnetic resonance imaging; NSAID, nonsteroidal anti-inflammatory drug. *Active inflammation compatible with sacroiliitis. †According to the modified New York criteria. Reproduced with permission from Rudwaleit et al. [7].

Classification criteria are developed to get a clear 'yes' or 'no' answer from a given patient, normally to decide on whether the patient would be suitable for a clinical study as patient populations need to be homogeneous for studies. In daily clinical practice such a clear decision is often not possible (and not always wanted), especially early in the course of the disease, and a more flexible approach is necessary. One possible diagnostic algorithm is shown in Figure 4.11 [33]. As the sensitivity and specificity for each of the parameters shown in this algorithm are known (Figure 4.12), the post-test probability for the diagnosis can be calculated if one or several of these parameters are positive. For this the pre-test probability that a patient with chronic back pain seen in primary care has axial SpA has to be known before any further details about clinical, laboratory or imaging parameters are available. As a result of the relatively low pre-test probability of about 5% (ie, 1 in 20 chronic back pain patients has axial SpA) [45], under these circumstances a combination of several clinical (such as inflammatory back pain, enthesitis, uveitis and peripheral arthritis), laboratory (such as HLA-B27 or C-reactive protein [CRP]) and imaging parameters (radiographs or MRI) are necessary for an early diagnosis.

Variables used in the ASAS criteria for classification of axial spondyloarthritis	
Clinical criterion	Definition
Inflammatory back pain	According to experts: four out of five of the following parameters present: (1) age at onset <40 years; (2) insidious onset; (3) improvement with exercise; (4) no improvement with rest; (5) pain at night (with improvement upon getting up)
Arthritis	Past or present active synovitis diagnosed by a doctor
Family history	Presence in first-degree or second-degree relatives of any of the following: (a) ankylosing spondylitis, (b) psoriasis (c) uveitis, (d) reactive arthritis, (e) inflammatory bowel disease
Psoriasis	Past or present psoriasis diagnosed by a doctor
Inflammatory bowel disease	Past or present Crohn's disease or ulcerative colitis diagnosed by a doctor
Dactylitis	Past or present dactylitis diagnosed by a doctor
Enthesitis	Heel enthesitis: past or present spontaneous pain or tenderness at examination of the site of the insertion of Achilles' tendon or plantar fascia at the calcaneus
Uveitis anterior	Past or present uveitis anterior, confirmed by an ophthalmologist
Good response to NSAIDs	24–48 hours after a full dose of a NSAID the back pain is not present anymore or much better
HLA-B27	Positive testing according to standard laboratory techniques
Elevated CRP	CRP above upper normal limit, in the presence of back pain, after exclusion of other causes for elevated CRP concentration
Sacroiliitis by radiographs	Bilateral grade 2–4 or unilateral grade 3–4, according to the modified New York criteria
Sacroiliitis by MRI	Active inflammatory lesions of sacroiliac joints with definite bone marrow oedema/ostitis suggestive of sacroilitis associated with spondyloarthritis

Figure 4.10 Variables used in the ASAS criteria for classification of axial spondyloarthritis. ASAS, Assessment in SpondyloArthritis international Society; CRP, C-reactive protein; HLA, human leukocyte antigen; MRI, magnetic resonance imaging; NSAID, nonsteroidal anti-inflammatory drug. Reproduced with permission from Rudwaleit et al. [7].

The more advanced the disease and the more chronic damage that has already occurred (such as syndesmophytes), the easier it is for a diagnosis to be made in the presence of just a few parameters (such as positive radiographs), but not early in the course of the disease. The algorithm shown in Figure 4.11 gives strong weight to inflammatory back pain as an entry criterion, although

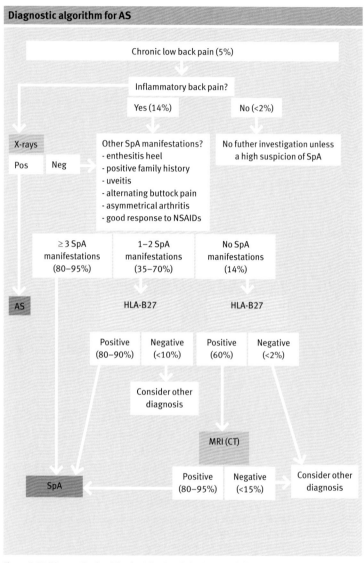

Figure 4.11 Diagnostic algorithm for AS. AS, ankylosing spondylitis; CT, computed tomography; HLA, human leukocyte antigen; MRI, magnetic resonance imaging; Pos, positive; Neg, negative; SpA, spondyloarthritis. Percentages indicate pre- or post-test probabilities. Reproduced with permission from Rudwaleit et al. [33].

Sensitivity, specificity and LR of AS and axial SpA features

	Sensitivity (%)	Specificity (%)	LR+
Inflammatory back pain	71–75	75–80	3.7
Enthesitis (heel pain)	16–37	89–94	3.4
Peripheral arthritis	40–62	90–98	4.0
Dactylitis	12–24	96–98	4.5
Anterior uveitis	10–22	97–99	7.3
Positive family history for SpA	7–36	93–99	6.4
Psoriasis	10–20	95–97	4.0
Inflammatory bowel disease	5–8	97–99	4.0
Good response to NSAIDs	61–77	80–85	5.1
Elevated acute phase reactants	38–69	67–80	2.5
HLA-B27 (axial involvement)	83–96	90–96	9.0
Magnetic resonance imaging (STIR)	90*	90*	9.0

Positive likelihood ratio (LR+) = sensitivity / (100 – specificity)

Figure 4.12 Sensitivity, specificity and LR of AS and axial SpA features. AS, ankylosing spondylitis; HLA, human leukocyte antigen; LR, likelihood ratio; NSAID, nonsteroidal anti-inflammatory drug; SpA, spondyloarthritis; STIR, short tau inversion recovery. *Best estimate. Reproduced with permission from Rudwaleit et al. [33].

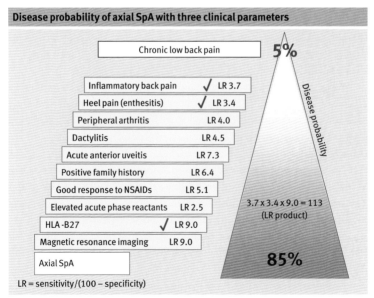

Figure 4.13 Disease probability of axial SpA with three clinical parameters. HLA, human leukocyte antigen; LR, likelihood ratio; NSAID, nonsteroidal anti-inflammatory drug; SpA, spondyloarthritis. Adapted from Rudwaleit et al. [4].

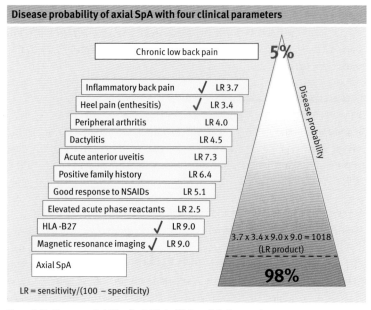

Figure 4.14 Disease probability of axial SpA with four clinical parameters.
HLA, human leukocyte antigen; LR, likelihood ratio; NSAID, nonsteroidal anti-inflammatory drug; SpA, spondyloarthritis. Adapted from Rudwaleit et al. [4].

the sensitivity for this symptom is not higher than 80%, so 20% of the patients with the disease would be missed if inflammatory back pain were regarded as essential.

Subsequently we proposed a slightly modified and even more flexible diagnostic approach [33]. If the sensitivity and specificity of a single parameter for a given disease (in this case axial SpA) are known, the likelihood ratio (LR) can be easily calculated (Figure 4.12), which is a good indicator for the diagnostic value of a parameter: the higher the LR, the higher the value of this parameter for diagnosis. If several parameters are present the LRs can be multiplied and the post-test probability calculated. Figures 4.13 and 4.14 give two examples of a combination of different SpA-typical parameters and the resulting post-test probability that a diagnosis of axial SpA is present, in the absence of radiographic sacroiliitis. As can be seen from the likelihood ratio values (Figures 4.12–4.14) a positive MRI and a positive HLA-B27 are the best single parameters in this diagnostic pyramid. The relevance of these two parameters, especially for early diagnosis, is also reflected in the ASAS classification criteria (see Figure 4.9) [7]. Using this approach in patients with chronic back pain, the clinical symptom of inflammatory back pain is one (important) clinical parameter, but it is not essential. Of note also, CRP has only a limited value in a diagnostic approach because of a relatively low sensitivity and even in a patient with active disease a positive CRP can be found in only about 60%.

Screening for axial SpA among patients with chronic back pain

In addition to establishing criteria for the classification and diagnosis of AS, screening strategies are of similar importance in alerting the primary care doctor to a diagnosis of inflammatory spine disease in patients with chronic back pain and when to refer these patients to the rheumatologist for a final diagnosis. Whether chronic back pain patients are first seen by primary care doctors, orthopaedists, physiotherapists or other doctors varies from country to country. Therefore, such strategies have to be adapted to the local conditions. Recently, we have proposed screening parameters for early referral of AS patients by primary care doctors that are easy to apply [46]. Such parameters have to be relatively sensitive and specific for the disease studied, easy to apply by non-specialists and should not be too expensive. We performed a study in the environs of Berlin, in Germany, asking all orthopaedists and primary care doctors to refer to an early axial SpA clinic patients with

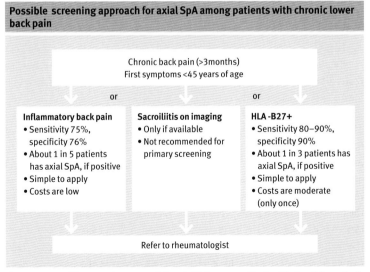

Possible screening approach for axial SpA among patients with chronic lower back pain

Chronic back pain (>3months)
First symptoms <45 years of age

or   or

Inflammatory back pain
- Sensitivity 75%, specificity 76%
- About 1 in 5 patients has axial SpA, if positive
- Simple to apply
- Costs are low

Sacroiliitis on imaging
- Only if available
- Not recommended for primary screening

HLA -B27+
- Sensitivity 80–90%, specificity 90%
- About 1 in 3 patients has axial SpA, if positive
- Simple to apply
- Costs are moderate (only once)

Refer to rheumatologist

Figure 4.15 Possible screening approach for axial SpA among patients with chronic lower back pain. HLA, human leukocyte antigen; SpA, spondyloarthritis. Adapted from Sieper et al. [46].

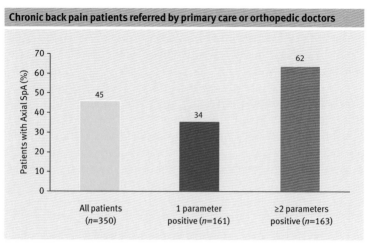

Figure 4.16 Chronic back pain patients referred from primary care or orthopaedic doctors. SpA, spondyloarthritis. Adapted from Brandt et al [47].

chronic back pain lasting for more than 3 months in whom the symptoms started at an age younger than 45, who fulfilled one or more of the following criteria: either fulfilling the clinical symptom of inflammatory back pain or being positive for HLA-B27, or showing evidence of sacroiliitis on imaging (Figure 4.15). Analysis of 350 referred patients showed that a final diagnosis of axial SpA could be made in about 45% of patients (Figure 4.16), half of whom had non-radiographic sacroiliitis [47]. These data clearly indicate that such a screening approach is feasible and effective, and that patients with non-radiographic axial SpA constitute a substantial part of the whole group of patients with axial SpA.

The value of HLA-B27 for screening and diagnosis of axial SpA

According to our calculations a final diagnosis of axial SpA can be made in one of three patients with chronic back pain (33%) who are positive for HLA-B27 [4, 46]. This implies that two of three patients do not have this diagnosis despite being positive for HLA-B27! This figure was also confirmed in a recent study [47]. In the past, many patients with back pain have been labelled as having AS, simply because they are positive for HLA-B27 and consequently many rheumatologists have been reluctant to use HLA-B27 in a diagnostic approach. However, if HLA-B27 is used together with other clinical and imaging parameters it is highly valuable in a diagnostic approach (see Figures 4.11–4.14) and as a screening tool. This is because of a relatively high sensitivity and specificity for HLA-B27, about 90% for both, and also because the test has to be performed just once in a lifetime (as a genetic marker there will be no change!) and gives a clear 'yes' or 'no' answer (about 5% false-negative or false-positive results are due to lab error), which is often much more difficult for the other SpA-typical parameters.

Chapter 5

Imaging in ankylosing spondylitis

Radiographs and magnetic resonance imaging (MRI) for sacroiliac (SI) joints and the spine are the most important imaging techniques for the diagnosis and follow-up of patients with spondyloarthritis (SpA), including response to treatment. If other sites outside the axial skeleton are affected they can also be investigated by these methods. In general, radiographs should not be performed more frequently than every 2 years because (chronic) changes occur slowly and investigations with MRI can be used more frequently, according to the clinical situation.

Radiographs

The investigation of SI joints and the spine by radiographs has been used since the 1930s for the diagnosis and staging of patients with AS. In contrast to MRI, radiographs can detect only chronic bony changes (damage) that are the consequence of inflammation and not inflammation itself. Therefore, radiographs are not suitable for early diagnosis of SpA, although they are still the method of choice for the detection of chronic changes and are widely used for diagnostic purposes in patients with already established disease (see modified New York criteria in Chapter 4). Erosive bony changes can also be detected early in the course of the disease by radiographs, although other methods such as computed tomography (CT) and MRI are superior for this. Radiographs are most important for the detection and follow-up of new bone formation, such as syndesmophytes in the spine.

Sacroiliac changes can be scored according to the grading discussed earlier in Chapter 4 which also shows examples of various grades of sacroiliitis (see Figures 4.3–4.5). Different approaches have been proposed for the radiological investigation of the SI joints with the intention of getting an optimal view of this irregularly shaped joint. None of them has been shown to be clearly superior. The Assessment in SpondyloArthritis international Society (ASAS) recommends performing radiographs of the whole pelvis because this allows assessment of the hip joints, as well as the SI joints; the hip joints are relatively frequently affected in spondyloarthritis. One possible differential diagnosis, osteitis condensans ilii, which can be found preferentially in middle-aged women, is shown in Figure 5.1.

Osteitis condensans ilii

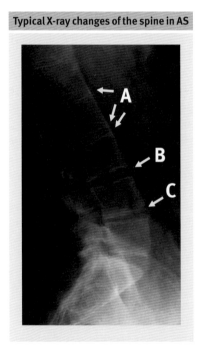

Figure 5.1 Osteitis condensans ilii. Radiograph of a woman aged 45 years with osteitis condensas ilii. The patient had low back pain for 3 months and was negative for HLA-B27. Figure provided courtesy of ASAS.

Typical X-ray changes of the spine in AS

Figure 5.2 Typical X-ray changes of the spine in AS. AS, ankylosing spondylitis. **(a)** bridging syndesmophytes; **(b)** erosion and sclerosis; **(c)** small syndesmophyte. Reproduced with permission from Baraliakos et al. [48].

When investigating the spine by radiographs, the cervical and lumbar spine should be included. Although changes in the thoracic spine are frequent, they are more difficult to detect because of the overlying lung tissue, so radiographs of the thoracic spine are not routinely assessed. Figure 5.2 shows typical spinal lesions that can be seen on radiographs: squaring of the vertebral body as a result of remodelling due to inflammation and new bone formation, sclerosis of the vertebral edges as a consequence of inflammation (shiny corners) and syndesmophytes. Syndesmophytes typically grow in a vertical direction whereas spondylophytes – typical for degenerative spine disease – grow in a horizontal direction (Figure 5.3). Figure 5.4 shows an example of an already ankylosed facet joint in a patient with AS. Figure 5.5 shows an AS patient with an Andersson II lesion (CT scan) resulting from a preceding spondylodisciitis with a subsequent insufficiency fracture at this site. Of note, osteoporosis of the spine as a consequence of local and systemic inflammation occurs more often in AS patients compared with age-matched controls, with increased risk for vertebral fractures, but not for non-vertebral fractures [49].

Figure 5.6 shows a radiograph from a patient with diffuse idiopathic skeletal hyperostosis (DISH; also known as Forestier disease), an important differential diagnosis of advanced AS. Note that the ligament in front of the vertebrae is ossified in combination with severe degenerative spinal changes, in the absence of AS-typical syndesmophytes. Radiographs of the SI joints are mostly normal although ossification of ligaments can imitate ankylosed SI joints.

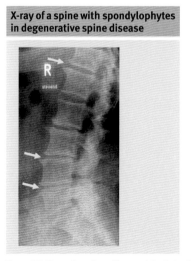

X-ray of a spine with spondylophytes in degenerative spine disease

Figure 5.3 **X-ray of a spine with spondylophytes in degenerative spine disease**.
Spondylophytes (arrows) are typical for degenerative spine disease and have a horizontal growth, while syndesmophytes (not shown here) show a vertical growth.

Facet joints ankylosed over time

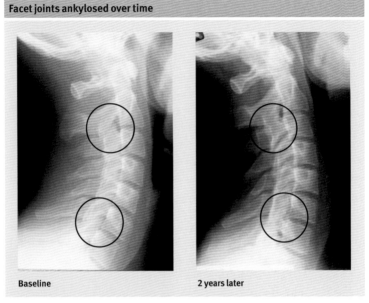

Baseline   2 years later

Figure 5.4 Facet joints ankylosed over time.

CT image showing Andersson II lesion in AS

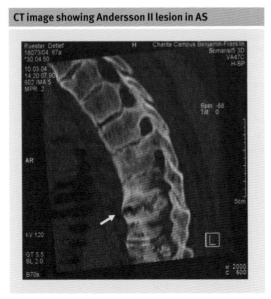

Figure 5.5 CT image showing Andersson II lesion in ankylosing spondylitis.
Spondylodisciitis with insufficiency fracture. Reproduced with permission from Sieper [50].

Diffuse idiopathic skeletal hyperostosis

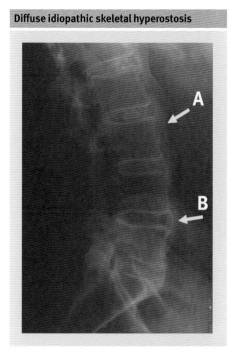

Figure 5.6 Diffuse idiopathic skeletal hyperostosis. Radiograph of a male patient aged 75 years with diffuse idiopathic skeletal hyperostosis who experienced chronic back pain. **(a)** ossification of ligament and no syndesmophytes; **(b)** spondylophytes.

Magnetic resonance imaging

MRI studies of the SI joints and the spine in SpA patients have made a major contribution in the last decade to a better understanding of the course of the disease, early diagnosis and use as an objective outcome measure for clinical trials.

Active inflammatory changes are best visualised by a fat-saturated, T2-weighted, turbo spin-echo sequence or a short tau inversion recovery (STIR) sequence with a high resolution that detects even minor fluid collections such as bone marrow oedema. Without fat saturation, fluid accumulation cannot be differentiated from fatty degeneration using this technique. Alternatively, administration of a paramagnetic contrast medium (gadolinium) detects increased perfusion (osteitis) in a T1-weighted sequence with fat saturation. These two sequences give largely overlapping information, although occasionally applying both methods can give additional value. Chronic changes such as fatty degeneration and erosions are best seen using a T1-weighted, turbo spin-echo sequence.

Active inflammatory sacroiliitis of the right joint by MRI

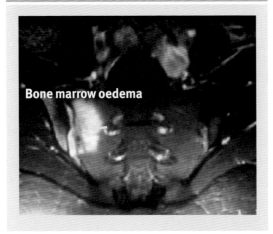

Bone marrow oedema

Figure 5.7 **Active inflammatory sacroiliitis of the right joint by MRI**. MRI, magnetic resonance imaging. STIR sequence.

MRI showing a patient with chronic sacroiliitis

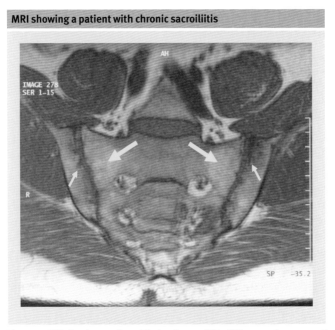

Figure 5.8 **MRI showing a patient with chronic sacroiliitis**. MRI, magnetic resonance image. Erosions (arrows) and fatty degeneration (bold arrows). T1-sequence.

The SI joints are imaged by MRI using a semicoronal section orientation along the long axis of the sacral bone. Typical active inflammatory lesions of the SI joints are: subchondral bone marrow oedema, capsulitis, synovitis and enthesitis. A typical example of an active sacroiliitis with subchondral bone marrow oedema is shown in Figure 5.7. The presence of just synovitis, capsulitis or enthesitis with no concomitant subchondral bone marrow oedema/osteitis is compatible with sacroiliitis but not sufficient to make a diagnosis of active sacroiliitis [51]. Possible differential diagnoses for an active inflammatory sacroiliitis in SpA are infectious sacroiliitis (typically also affecting the surrounding soft tissue), fracture of the ileum bone or the sacrum bone, and bone tumour. T1-weighted sequences can detect chronic changes such as erosions and fatty degeneration which are early signs of chronic damage (Figure 5.8).

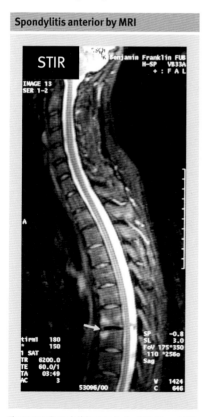

Spondylitis anterior by MRI

Figure 5.9 Spondylitis anterior by MRI. Spondylitis anterior (arrow) with active inflammation.

An efficient spinal imaging protocol comprises a sagittal, T1-weighted, turbo spin-echo sequence and a sagittal, fat-saturated, T2-weighted turbo spin-echo or STIR sequence with high resolution. Coronal slices of the entire spine may be used for better assessment of the costovertebral and costotransverse joints and the facet joints. Some examples of active inflammation of the spine in patients with axial SpA are shown in the following figures: spondylitis anterior (Figure 5.9), spondylitis posterior (Figure 5.10) and spondylodisciitis (Figure 5.11).

Active spondylitis posterior by MRI

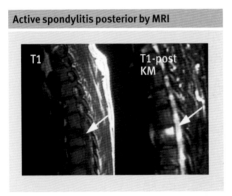

Figure 5.10 Active spondylitis posterior by MRI. MRI, magnetic resonance imaging. Reproduced with permission from Braun et al. [52].

Spondylodisciitis by MRI in axial spondyloarthritis

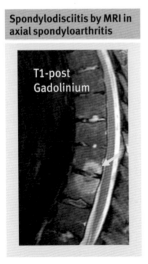

Figure 5.11 Spondylodisciitis by MRI in axial spondyloarthritis. MRI, magnetic resonance imaging. Figure provided courtesy of KG Hermann, Berlin, Germany.

An important and sometimes difficult differential diagnosis is erosive osteochondritis (Figure 5.12) as a consequence of degenerative disc disease, which resembles the spondylodisciitis seen in SpA patients. These lesions are most often located in the lumbar spine and patients would normally have no other features typical for AS/SpA and normal SI joints. T1-weighted sequences can also detect chronic changes such as erosions and fatty degeneration – similar to the SI joints – in the spine of patients with axial SpA.

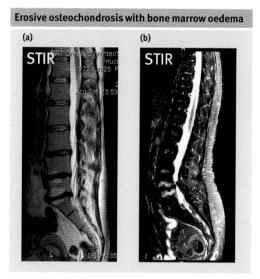

Figure 5.12 Erosive osteochondrosis with bone marrow oedema. (a) early case with oedema but without major erosions; **(b)** more advanced case with oedema and erosions.

Other imaging techniques

Scintigraphy has been used for many decades for the detection of active inflammation in SpA patients. However, it no longer plays a role in the diagnosis and management of SpA patients because of limited sensitivity and specificity and has been replaced by MRI [53]. Chronic bony changes can be better detected by CT (Figure 5.13) rather than radiographs. However, CT is rarely used because of a much higher radiation exposure. Active inflammatory changes cannot be seen by CT and fatty degeneration of the bone marrow, as an early sign of chronic change, is detectable only by MRI and not by CT.

For a more detailed description of imaging in AS, including its early forms, see also the ASAS handbook on assessment of spondyloarthritis [51].

Sacroiliitis grade II bilaterally on computed tomography

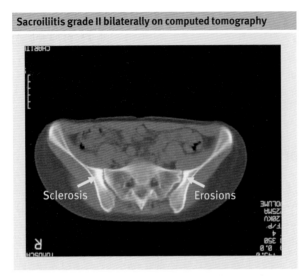

Figure 5.13 Sacroiliitis grade II bilaterally on computed tomography.

Chapter 6

Management of ankylosing spondylitis

Recently, the Assessment of SpondyloArthritis international Society (ASAS) and European League Against Rheumatism (EULAR) recommendations on the management of AS have been published, based on a thorough analysis of the available literature and on a meeting of spondyloarthritides (SpA) experts. These recommendations are shown in Figures 6.1 and 6.2 [54]. Non-drug approaches are part of the therapy at all stages of the disease. For the predominantly axial manifestation, the treatment options are limited to non-steroidal anti-inflammatory drugs (NSAIDs) as a kind of basic treatment, followed by tumour necrosis factor (TNF)-blocker therapy if this conventional treatment fails. If the clinical picture is dominated by peripheral symptoms such as arthritis or enthesitis, treatment with sulfasalazine and/or local steroid injection should be tried first before TNF blockers are considered.

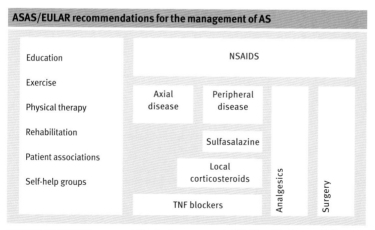

Figure 6.1 ASAS/EULAR recommendations for the management of AS. AS, ankylosing spondylitis; ASAS, Assessment in SpondyloArthritis international Society; EULAR, European League Against Rheumatism; NSAID, nonsteroidal anti-inflammatory drug. Reproduced with permission from Zochling et al. [54].

ASAS/EULAR recommendations for the management of AS

1. The treatment of AS should be tailored according to: the current manifestations of the disease (axial, peripheral, entheseal, extraarticular symptoms and signs), the level of current symptoms, clinical findings, and prognostic indicators, disease activity/ inflammation, pain, function, disability, handicap, structural damage, hip involvement, spinal deformities, the general clinical status (age, gender, comorbidity, concomitant medications, the wishes and expectations of the patient.

2. The disease monitoring of AS patients should include: patient history (eg, questionnaires), clinical parameters, laboratory tests, and imaging, all according to the clinical presentation as well as the ASAS core set. The frequency of monitoring should be decided on an individual basis depending on symptoms, severity and medication.

3. The optimal management of AS requires a combination of non-pharmacological and pharmacological treatment modalities.

4. Non-pharmacological therapy of AS should include patient education and regular exercise. Individual and group physical therapy should be considered. Patient associations and self help groups may be useful.

5. NSAIDs are recommended as first-line drug therapy for AS patients with pain and stiffness. In those with increased gastrointestinal risk, non-selective NSAIDs plus a gastro-protective agent, or a selective COX-2 inhibitor could be used.

6. Analgesics, such as paracetamol and opioids, might be considered for pain control in patients in whom NSAIDs are insufficient, contraindicated, and/or poorly tolerated.

7. Corticosteroid injections directed to the local site of musculoskeletal inflammation may be considered. The use of systemic corticosteroids for axial disease is not supported by evidence.

8. There is no evidence for the usefulness of DMARDs, including sulfasalazine and methotrexate, to treat axial disease. Sulfasalazine may be considered in patients with peripheral arthritis.

9. Anti-TNF therapy should be given to patients with persistently high disease activity and failure of other treatments according to the ASAS recommendations. There is no evidence for an obligatory use of DMARDs prior to or concomitant with anti-TNF therapy in patients with axial disease.

10. Joint replacement has to be considered in patients with radiographic evidence of advanced hip involvement who have refractory pain and disability, even in young patients. Spinal surgery is useful in selected patients.

Figure 6.2 ASAS/EULAR recommendations for the management of AS. AS, ankylosing spondylitis; ASAS, Assessment in SpondyloArthritis international Society; COX-2, cyclooxygenase 2; DMARD, disease-modifying anti-rheumatic drugs; EULAR, European League Against Rheumatism; NSAID, nonsteroidal anti-inflammatory drug; TNF, tumour necrosis factor. Reproduced with permission from Zochling et al. [54].

Non-drug treatment

Physiotherapy is the most important non-pharmacological aspect of AS management and was for a long time the most important. Its primary aims are to prevent and/or reduce restriction of spinal mobility and the development of disability, and to improve the symptoms of pain and stiffness. Once the diagnosis has been made the patient should be referred to a physical therapist who will teach the patient the exercises that he or she should perform regularly. As the main long-term outcome that should be prevented is a flexion deformity of the spine, exercises concentrate on extension and rotation of the spine. An exercise sequence for AS patients is shown in Figure 6.3.

Patients should be advised to exercise daily at home and to attend weekly group physical therapy. The patient's own efforts are the key to future success and the AS patient has to be convinced that a daily exercise programme should become a normal part of the day. In the long-term, many patients do not need regular prescriptions; however, there should be some mechanisms in place to ensure that the patient is seen and assessed regularly by the physical therapist. If patients are symptomatic and complain about pain or stiffness, they should be treated in addition with NSAIDs (see below) or other effective drugs to permit full mobilization during the exercises. These exercises should be continued regularly lifelong. Furthermore, patients should be encouraged to participate in moderate sport activities such as swimming and cycling.

Patient education is an essential part of non-pharmacological therapy and should include information about pathogenesis, clinical manifestations and course of the disease, physiotherapy and ergotherapy, how to cope with the disease, and counselling about the socioeconomic consequences of the disease. Patients should also be encouraged to get engaged in patient associations and patient self-help groups.

Drug treatment

NSAID treatment

The NSAIDs are still regarded as the cornerstone of pharmacological intervention for AS with a good anti-inflammatory capacity, reducing pain and stiffness rapidly after 48–72 hours [55, 56]. Most AS patients report a good or very good efficacy when treated with a full dose of an NSAID, in contrast to patients with chronic back pain from other causes (Figure 6.4). Figure 6.5 shows NSAIDs that are used for the treatment of AS [56]. The dosing should be adjusted to the clinical symptoms and the half-life of the drug: normally the effect of the drug should cover the night and the early morning (ie, morning stiffness); however, often

Physical therapy for patients with AS

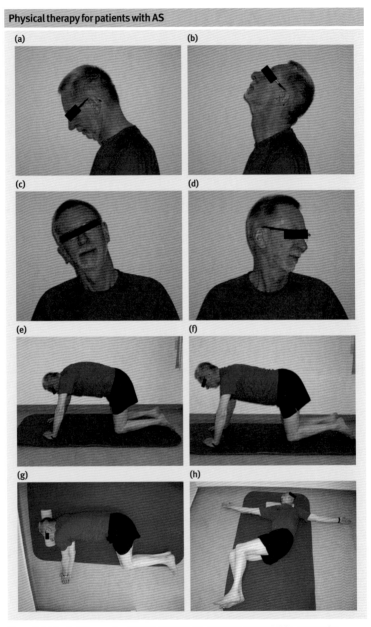

Figure 6.3 Physical therapy for patients with AS. AS, ankylosing spondylitis. An exercise sequence used in ankylosing spondylitis. Cervical spine exercises include: **(a)** full flexion; **(b)** extension; **(c)** lateral flexion; and **(d)** rotation. A sequence of **(e)** back flexion; and **(f)** extension is followed by rotation in a lying position **(g–h)**.

Physical therapy for patients with AS (cont'd)

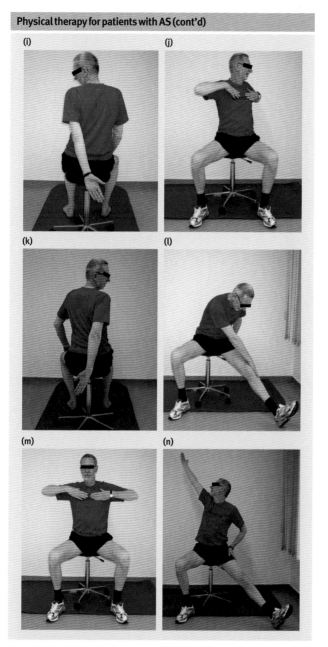

Figure 6.3 Physical therapy for patients with AS (cont'd). AS, ankylosing spondylitis. A sequence of rotations in a sitting position **(i–n)**. Finally, breathing is practiced using the thoracic muscles (not shown).

Efficacy of NSAIDs for the treatment of patients with AS

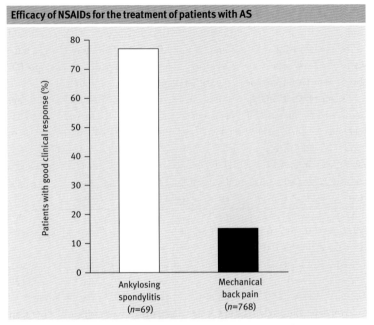

Figure 6.4 Efficacy of NSAIDs for the treatment of patients with AS. AS, ankylosing spondylitis; NSAID, nonsteroidal anti-inflammatory drug. Adapted from Amor et al. [57].

Dosage of NSAIDs used in the treatment of patients with AS

Drug	Half-life (hours)	Approved maximum daily dosage (mg)†
Aceclofenac	about 4	200
Celecoxib	8–12	400
Diclofenac*	about 2	150
Etoricoxib	about 22	90
Ibuprofen	1.8–3.5	2400
Indomethacin*	about 2	150
Ketoprofen	1.5–2.5	200
Meloxicam	about 20	15
Naproxen	10–18	1000
Piroxicam	30–60	20
Phenylbutazone	50–100	600

Figure 6.5 NSAID therapy in patients with AS. AS, ankylosing spondylitis; NSAID, nonsteroidal anti-inflammatory drug. *slow-release formula available †normally for arthritis. Reproduced with permission from Song et al. [56].

24-hour treatment is necessary. Phenylbutazone, which has been approved for short-term treatment, is probably one of the most effective NSAIDs, but should be reserved for patients in whom other NSAIDs failed and should be given for only a few days, because of possible bone marrow toxicity. At least two NSAIDs should have been tested before NSAID treatment failure is assumed.

Frequently patients are not treated with a full dose of NSAIDs and/or are not treated continuously despite being symptomatic. A major reason for this is that both patients and treating doctors are often concerned about the toxicity of continuous NSAID treatment [58]. We have recently summarized and discussed the benefits and risks of NSAID treatment in AS. Besides good efficacy for signs and symptoms there is even evidence that continuous therapy with NSAIDs might stop the new formation of syndesmophytes in the spine, as reported recently [59]. It is not clear at the moment whether such an effect can be explained by the suppression of inflammation or, whether by direct inhibition of osteoblast activity by NSAIDs, through the suppression of prostaglandins.

There are now sufficient data available on the risks of long-term treatment with NSAIDs in several large non-AS trials: the probability in patients younger than 60 years and with no gastrointestinal (GI) or cardiovascular (CV) comorbidities is 1% or less of developing serious GI or CV side effects when treated with a full dose of an NSAID for 1 year. Also the risk for renal and liver side effects is known and seems to be acceptable [56]. Thus, when AS patients are active, they should be treated with a sufficient, and if necessary continuous, dose of NSAIDs. Patients should be informed about and monitored for potential toxicity both before and during treatment.

Simple analgesics such as paracetamol and opioids have at most a limited role in the treatment of AS and are used in patients who have contraindications to treatment with NSAIDs and/or a TNF blocker.

Corticosteroids and DMARDS

There is no clear role for systemic corticosteroids in the treatment of AS because a high dose is normally necessary to achieve a measurable clinical improvement. In case of inflammation at single joints, such as a sacroiliac (SI) joint or peripheral joint, local steroid injections have proved effective [60].

Conventional disease-modifying anti-rheumatic drugs (DMARDs) play a dominant role in the treatment of rheumatoid arthritis, but they have no proven efficacy for the axial manifestations of AS. Figure 6.6 summarizes three studies with sulfazalazine, leflunomide and methotrexate in AS, clearly showing that there is no improvement in the disease activity in these patients [61–63]. DMARDs have a limited efficacy for the peripheral manifestations in AS; the best data are available for sulfasalazine given at a dose of 2–3 g/day orally [64].

Conventional DMARDs are not effective for the treatment of AS

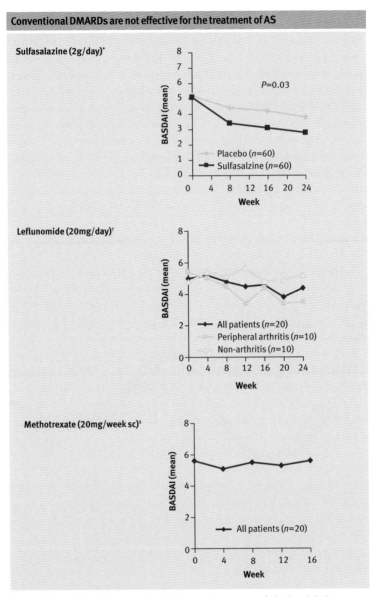

Figure 6.6 Conventional DMARDs are not effective for the treatment of AS. AS, ankylosing spondylitis; BASDAI, Bath Ankylosing Spondylitis Disease Activity Index; DMARD, disease-modifying anti-rheumatic drugs. Data from [*]Braun J et al. [65]; [†]Haibel et al. [61]; [‡]Haibel et al. [66].

Anti-TNF-α-blocking agents

It can be estimated that about 20% of AS patients are still active despite optimal treatment with NSAIDs. This means that the demonstration of good or very good efficacy of TNF blockers in the treatment of patients with active AS can be regarded as a breakthrough in the therapy of these AS patients. These drugs not only improve signs and symptoms rapidly and in a high percentage of patients, but also normalize acute phase reactants and reduce acute inflammation in SI joints and the spine as shown by magnetic resonance imaging (MRI). Currently there are three biologic agents targeting TNF-α which have been approved for the treatment of AS (Figure 6.7) [67].

Dosage of TNF-blocking agents in the treatment of AS		
Drug	**AS**	**Application**
Infliximab	5 mg/kg	i.v. at week 0, 2, 6, Every 6–8 weeks
Etanercept	25 mg	s.c. twice weekly
	50 mg	s.c. once weekly
Adalimumab	40 mg	s.c. every 2 weeks

Figure 6.7 Dosage of TNF-blocking agents in the treatment of AS. AS, ankylosing spondylitis; TNF, tumour necrosis factor.

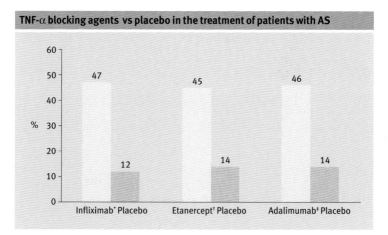

Figure 6.8 TNF-α blocking agents vs placebo in the treatment of patients with AS.
AS, ankylosing spondylitis; TNF, tumour necrosis factor. Response to treatment at 24 weeks was defined using ASAS response criteria 40 (ie, 40% improvement from baseline). Data from *van der Heijde et al. [68]; †Davis et al. [70]; ‡van der Heijde et al. [69]. Figure provided courtesy of ASAS.

All three TNF-blocking agents have a similar efficacy on rheumatic symptoms: about half the patients reach a 50% improvement in their disease activity as measured by the Bath Ankylosing Spondylitis Disease Activity Index (BASDAI) or a 40% improvement in the Assessment of SpondyloArthritis international Society (ASAS) composite outcome score (Figure 6.8) [69, 71, 72]. These patients had a high disease activity before despite being on optimal treatment with NSAIDs. The ASAS clinical outcome criteria, which are used in all AS and SpA trials, are shown in Figures 6.9–6.11 [55, 67].

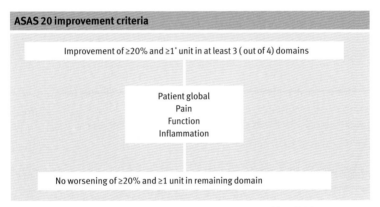

Figure 6.9 ASAS 20 improvement criteria. ASAS, Assessment in SpondyloArthritis international Society. *On a numerical rating scale (0–10). A visual analogue scale (0–100) can also be used. Data from Anderson et al. [55].

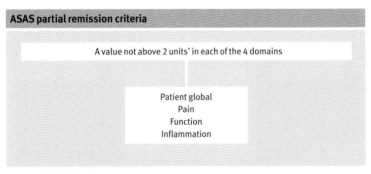

Figure 6.10 ASAS partial remission criteria. ASAS, Assessment in SpondyloArthritis international Society. *On a numerical rating scale (0–10). A visual analogue scale (0–100) can also be used. Data from Anderson et al. [55].

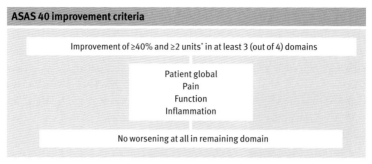

ASAS 40 improvement criteria

Improvement of ≥40% and ≥2 units* in at least 3 (out of 4) domains

Patient global
Pain
Function
Inflammation

No worsening at all in remaining domain

Figure 6.11 ASAS 40 improvement criteria. ASAS, Assessment in SpondyloArthritis international Society. *On a numerical rating scale (0–10). A visual analogue scale (0–100) can also be used. Reproduced with permission from Brandt et al. [67].

Most recently, a new ankylosing spondylitis disease activity index has been proposed by ASAS which includes, besides clinical parameters, C-reactive protein (CRP) and which performed best in a retrospective analysis of clinical cohorts and treatment trials (Figures 6.12–6.13) [73].

AS disease activity score I

Parameters used for the calculation of the AS disease activity score

1. Total back pain (BASDAI question 2)

2. Patient global (on a scale 0–10)

3. Peripheral pain/swelling (BASDAI question 3)

4. Duration of morning stiffness (BASDAI question 6)

5. C-reactive protein in mg/l (or erythrocyte sedimentation rate)

Figure 6.12 AS disease activity score I. AS, ankylosing spondylitis; BASDAI, Bath Ankylosing Spondylitis Disease Activity Index. Data from van der Heijde et al. [73].

AS disease activity score II calculation

ASDAS$_{CRP}$

$0.121 \times$ total + $0.110 \times$ patient + $0.073 \times$ peripheral + $0.058 \times$ duration + $0.579 \times \mathrm{Ln(CRP+1)}$
back pain   global   pain/swelling   of morning stiffness

ASDAS$_{ESR}$

$0.113 \times$ patient + $0.293 \times \sqrt{ESR}$ + $0.086 \times$ peripheral + $0.069 \times$ duration of + $0.079 \times$ total
global   pain/swelling   morning stiffness   back pain

The ASDAS$_{CRP}$ is the preferred ASDAS but the ASDAS$_{ESR}$ can be used in case CRP is not available. CRP in mg/l; all patient assessments are on a 10 cm scale.

Figure 6.13 AS disease activity score II. ASDAS, ankylosing spondylitis disease activity score; CRP, C-reactive protein; ESR, erythrocyte sedimentation rate. Data from van der Heijde et al. [73].

Impressive reduction of inflammatory lesions either in the SI joints or in the spine have been demonstrated for all three TNF blockers (Figures 6.14–6.17) [74–76].

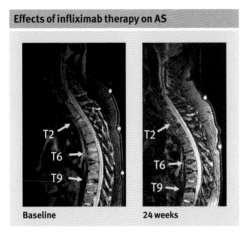

Effects of infliximab therapy on AS

Baseline   24 weeks

Figure 6.14 **Effects of infliximab therapy on AS**. AS, ankylosing spondylitis. MRI images of the thoracic vertebrae of a patient with AS at baseline and after 24 weeks of infliximab therapy. Reproduced with permission from Braun et al. [74].

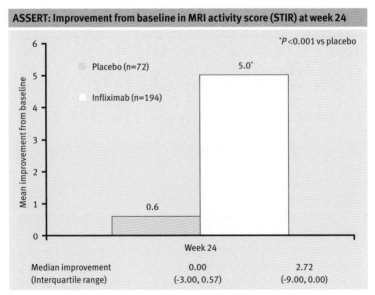

ASSERT: Improvement from baseline in MRI activity score (STIR) at week 24

Median improvement	0.00	2.72
(Interquartile range)	(-3.00, 0.57)	(-9.00, 0.00)

Figure 6.15 **ASSERT: Improvement from baseline in MRI activity score (STIR) at week 24**. ASSERT, Ankylosing Spondylitis Study for the Evaluation of Recombinant infliximab Therapy; MRI, magnetic resonance image. Data from Braun et al. [74].

Sacroiliac joints before and after etanercept treatment

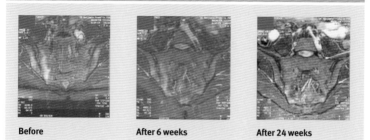

Before　　　　　　　**After 6 weeks**　　　　　　　**After 24 weeks**

Figure 6.16 Sacroiliac joints before and after etanercept treatment. Reproduced with permission from Rudwaleit et al. [75].

Adalimumab reduces inflammation in the spine of a patient with AS

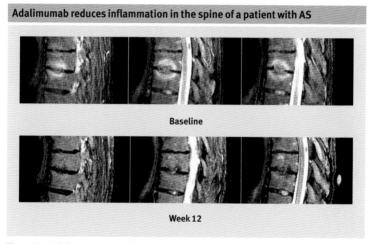

Baseline

Week 12

Figure 6.17 Adalimumab reduces inflammation in the spine of a patient with AS.
AS, ankylosing spondylitis. Reproduced with permission from Lambert et al. [76].

Interestingly, there is still a further decrease of inflammation if patients are treated over 2 years, although in a small proportion of patients inflammation, as seen by MRI, is not suppressed completely [77]. AS and related SpA seem to be the disease for which TNF blockers are most effective, probably more effective than in rheumatoid arthritis [78]. Long-term follow-up of AS patients treated with TNF blockers (Figures 6.18 and 6.19) has to date been published for up to 7 years, showing good long-term efficacy if treatment is continued [79]. A drop-out rate of about 10% per year can be expected for patients on long-term treatment, for various reasons such as side effects, loss of efficacy or lack of compliance. However, when treatment was stopped, nearly all these patients with long-standing active disease showed a flare-up. It still has to be seen whether this is the case when patients are treated earlier.

Although TNF-blocker treatment of active inflammation of the SI joint or spine is very effective in AS, as shown by MRI, the growth of syndesmophytes in the spine, as seen by radiographs, could not be completely stopped over a treatment period of 2 years with infliximab, etanercept or adalimumab (presented at the American College of Radiology meeting in 2008) [80, 81]. As shown in Figure 2.8, which outlined the proposed sequence of structural damage in AS, new bone formation such as growth of syndesmophytes is a type of repair mechanism for damaged cartilage/bone [26, 27]. Thus, when TNF-blocker therapy starts before erosive damage has occurred new bone formation can probably also be prevented. However, if there are already erosions, TNF blockers have no effect on subsequent ossification because they do not inhibit osteoblasts. Following this reasoning, it can be speculated that early treatment with TNF blockers is the most effective way to prevent syndesmophytes and ankylosis in the long-term. This has to be proven by future studies. Furthermore, the observed small growth of syndesmophytes is probably clinically not meaningful, because it has been shown that in the same patients function and spinal mobility improved over 2 years of treatment [79, 82].

In contrast to the treatment of rheumatoid arthritis, there is no evidence that combination of a TNF blocker with a conventional DMARD is superior compared with treatment of AS with a TNF blocker alone. Most of the patients in the studies were indeed treated with TNF-blocker monotherapy. Two recent studies comparing infliximab alone versus infliximab plus methotrexate showed clearly that there was no significant difference between the two groups regarding efficacy and side effects [83, 84].

Extrarheumatic manifestations or comorbidities such as uveitis, psoriasis or inflammatory bowel disease (IBD) are present or have occurred in the past in 40–50% of AS patients, as discussed earlier [36]. Thus, it is also interesting whether the three TNF blockers differ in their efficacy with regard to these manifestations. Both monoclonal antibodies have been shown to be effective for the treatment of Crohn's disease, and infliximab for ulcerative colitis, whereas etanercept does not work in IBD. When it was investigated whether TNF blockers reduce flares or a new onset of IBD in AS patients treated for their rheumatic manifestations, infliximab was clearly superior to etanercept whereas the number of patients treated with adalimumab was too small in this meta-analysis to allow any further conclusions [85]. In another meta-analysis of

Efficacy of TNF-antagonists in patients with AS

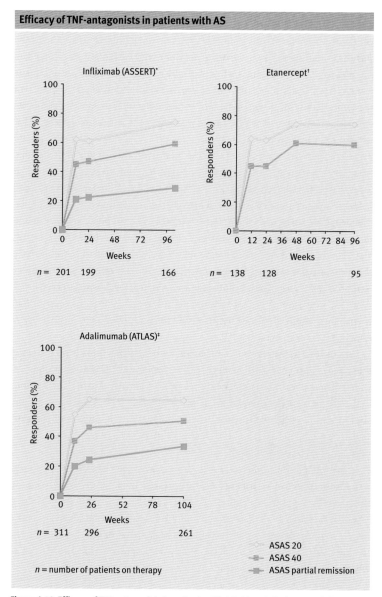

Figure 6.18 Efficacy of TNF-antagonists in patients with AS. AS, ankylosing spondylitis. ASAS, Assessment in SpondyloArthritis international Society; TNF, tumour necrosis factor. Data from *Braun et al. [79]; †Davis et al. [70]; ‡van der Heijde et al. [86]. Figure provided courtesy of ASAS.

trials from AS patients treated with TNF blockers both infliximab and etanercept reduced flares of uveitis, but infliximab was slightly more effective [87]. Based on data from a small retrospective study and from one large but uncontrolled observational study, adalimumab seems also to reduce flares of uveitis, from 15 flares per 100 patient-years before treatment to 7.4 in one of the studies [88]. All three TNF blockers are effective for psoriasis, although infliximab shows the best efficacy on the skin in the doses normally used for the treatment of AS.

Anti-TNF therapy in the treatment of juvenile spondyloarthritis

The first symptoms of AS occur in 15–20% of cases before the age of 20 years and juvenile and adult spondyloarthritis should be seen as one disease with a continuum. While the juvenile forms normally present first with a predominance of peripheral manifestations (enthesitis and peripheral arthritis), many of the juvenile patients later develop the full picture of typical AS. Both infliximab and etanercept have shown good efficacy in patients with juvenile SpA or enthesitis-related arthritis in smaller studies; studies with adalimumab are ongoing for this indication.

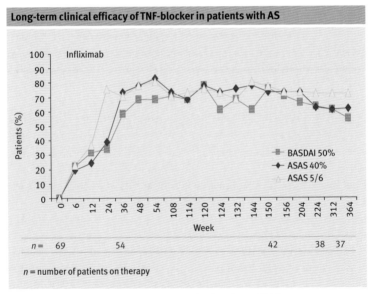

Figure 6.19 Long-term clinical efficacy of TNF-blocker in patients with AS.
ASAS, Assessment in SpondyloArthritis international Society; Bath Ankylosing Spondylitis Disease Activity Index. Adapted from Braun et al. [71]; Braun et al. [89]; Baraliakos et al. [90].

Adverse events of anti-TNF therapy

The adverse events in AS patients treated with TNF blockers do not differ from those seen in other diseases such as rheumatoid arthritis and Crohn's disease. However, AS patients are normally younger and have been less frequently treated with glucocorticoids or immunosuppressive drugs compared with the other two diseases. Thus, the number and the severity of side effects can be expected to be at least no higher than for other chronic inflammatory diseases, but possibly even lower. Comparative data on this are not available at this time, but application and implementation of the usual precautions and contraindications for biologic therapy should be followed, especially screening for latent tuberculosis (TB) before anti-TNF therapy is initiated.

According to most national guidelines a patient's history should be taken, a radiograph of the chest performed and immune response to TB tested either by tuberculin skin test and/or an in vitro T-cell assay for TB-specific antigens. Normally, patients are treated with 300 mg isoniazide for 9 months or alternatively with 600 mg rifampicin for 4–6 months before the start of TNF-blocker therapy. Other infections including opportunistic infections can occur in a small percentage of patients. In rheumatoid arthritis cohorts (any) infections were about twice as high in TNF-blocker-treated patients compared with patients on conventional therapy. A small increase in the risk of developing lymphoproliferative disorders cannot be excluded at this stage, allergic reactions occur, and the occurrence of neurological events and congestive heart failure has been reported occasionally.

Which patients should be treated with TNF blockers?

International recommendations for the initiation of anti-TNF-α therapy in patients with AS were developed and published by ASAS based on a review of published reports and a consensus meeting of international experts [54]. These recommendations are shown in Figures 6.20–6.22. Discontinuation of anti-TNF-α therapy should be strongly considered in non-responders after 12 weeks' treatment (Figure 6.22). Response is defined as: (1) improvement of at least 50% or 2 units (on a 0–10 scale) of the BASDAI in addition to (2) an expert opinion that treatment should be continued, again not just relying on patients' subjective symptoms.

Similar recommendations or guidelines have been published by national societies such as the British Society for Rheumatology (Figure 6.23) the Canadian Rheumatology Association (Figure 6.24), and the Spondylitis Association of America (Figure 6.25), following the reasoning of the ASAS recommendations, only with slight modifications [91, 92].

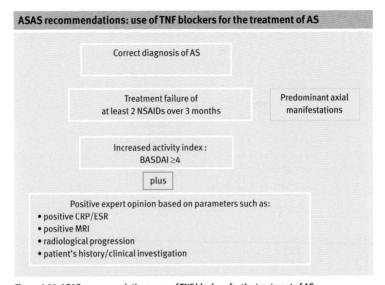

Figure 6.20 ASAS recommendations: use of TNF blockers for the treatment of AS.
AS, ankylosing spondylitis; ASAS, Assessment in SpondyloArthritis international Society.
BASDAI, Bath Ankylosing Spondylitis Disease Activity Index; CRP, C-reactive protein; ESR,
erythrocyte sedimentation rate; MRI, magnetic resonance imaging; NSAID, nonsteroidal anti-
inflammatory drug; TNF, tumour necrosis factor. Data from Braun et al. [93].

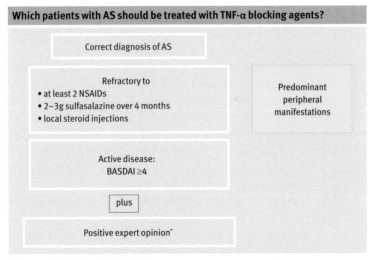

Figure 6.21 Which patients with AS should be treated with TNF-α blocking agents?
AS, ankylosing spondylitis. BASDAI, Bath Ankylosing Spondylitis Disease Activity Index;
NSAID, nonsteroidal anti-inflammatory drug; TNF, tumour necrosis factor. *See Figure 6.20.
Data from Braun et al. [93].

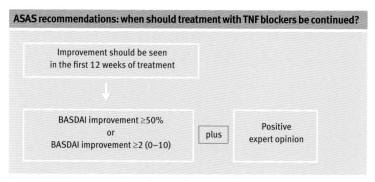

Figure 6.22 ASAS recommendations: when should treatment with TNF blockers be continued?
ASAS, Assessment in SpondyloArthritis international Society. BASDAI, Bath Ankylosing
Spondylitis Disease Activity Index; TNF, tumour necrosis factor. Data from Braun et al. [93].

British Society for Rheumatology guidelines for prescribing TNF blockers in the treatment of AS

- Diagnosis
  - Modified New York criteria

- Disease activity
  - BASDAI at least 4 (scale 0–10)
  - And spinal pain (VAS 0–10) at least 4 cm
  - Both on two occasions at least 4 weeks apart without any change of treatment

- Previous treatment
  - Failure of conventional treatment with two or more NSAIDs, each taken sequentially at maximum tolerated/recommended dosage for 4 weeks

- Criteria for withdrawal
  - Development of severe side effects
  - Inefficacy, as indicated by failure of the BASDAI to improve by 50% or to fall at least 2 units and/or for the spinal pain VAS to reduce by at least 2 units after 3 months

**Figure 6.23 British Society for Rheumatology guidelines for prescribing TNF blockers
in the treatment of AS.** AS, ankylosing spondylitis; BASDAI, Bath Ankylosing Spondylitis
Disease Activity Index; NSAID, nonsteroidal anti-inflammatory drug; TNF, tumour necrosis
factor; VAS, visual analogue scale. Adapted from Keat et al. [91].

The Canadian Rheumatology Association recommendations for the treatment of AS with TNF-blockers

• Anti-TNF treatment should be given under supervision of a rheumatologist

• Failure of conventional treatment
 – At least 3 NSAIDs, each administered over a minimum 2-week period at accepted maximum dosage if tolerated
 – There is no evidence to support the obligatory use of DMARDs before or together with TNF-blockers
 – Sulfasalazine and/or methotrexate might be considered in patients with peripheral arthritis

• Disease activity (at least 2 of the following)
 – BASDAI >4
 – Elevated CRP and/or ESR
 – Inflammatory lesions in the sacroiliac joint and/or spine on MRI

• Responder criteria
 – Reduction of BASDAI by 2 (0–10) or a relative reduction of 50% after 16 weeks

Figure 6.24 The Canadian Rheumatology Association recommendations for the treatment of AS with TNF-blockers. AS, ankylosing spondylitis; BASDAI, Bath Ankylosing Spondylitis Disease Activity Index; CRP, C-reactive protein; DMARD, disease-modifying anti-rheumatic drug; ESR, erythrocyte sedimentation rate; MRI magnetic resonance imaging; NSAID, nonsteroidal anti-inflammatory drug; TNF, tumour necrosis factor. Adapted from Maksymowych et al. [92].

Prognostic parameters in ankylosing spondylitis

When an analysis was made of which parameters predict a response to TNF blockers best, short disease duration and/or young age were the best predictors, indicating that patients with long-lasting disease also have causes other than inflammation contributing to the clinical symptoms [94, 95]. An elevated CRP and active inflammation, as shown by MRI, were also predictive, although not as good as short disease duration and young age [96].

In general, AS is a slowly progressing disease. In patients with a mean disease duration of about 20 years, syndesmophytes of the spine were detectable only in about 60% [34]. A growth of syndesmophytes is normally visible on radiographs only over a follow-up period of at least 2 years. However, there is a subgroup of still ill-defined patients who suffer from a more rapid progression. An older retrospective study reported the presence of hip arthritis, elevated erythrocyte sedimentation rate, young age at onset, poor response to NSAID treatment and extraspinal manifestations as predictors of a more severe course [97]. In more recent studies, the presence of syndesmophytes at baseline was the best predictor for the development of more syndesmophytes [34].

The Spondylitis Association of America guidelines for the use of anti-TNF therapy in patients with AS

- Diagnosis: modified New York criteria

- Disease activity
  - BASDAI ≥4 (scale 0–10)
  - Physician global assessment of ≥2 on a Likert scale: 0=none, 1=mild, 2=moderate, 3=severe, 4=very severe

- Failure of previous treatment
  - Failure by lack of response or intolerability to ≥2 NSAIDs for at least 3 months for all 3 presentations: axial, peripheral arthritis, enthesitis
  - Patients with peripheral arthritis must have had a lack of response to >1 DMARD (sulfasalazine preferred). Not required for axial disease or enthesitis (steroid injection not required)

- Dosing
  - Etanercept 2x25 mg sq twice a week (note from the authors: a dosing of 50 mg sq once a week was not yet available when these recommendations were published)
  - Infliximab 5 mg /kg IV every 6–8 weeks
  - Adalimumab (note from the authors: this drug was not yet approved when these recommendations were published; normal dosing: 40 mg sq every 2 weeks)

- Responder criteria
  - Improvement of BASDAI by at least 2 units and Physician's Global >1

- Time of evaluation
  - 6–8 weeks

- Tuberculosis precautions
  - Tuberculosis screening and treatment as indicated by the American Thoracic Association

Figure 6.25 The Spondylitis Association of America guidelines for the use of anti-TNF therapy in patients with AS. AS, ankylosing spondylitis; BASDAI, Bath Ankylosing Spondylitis Disease Activity Index; DMARD, disease-modifying anti-rheumatic drugs; NSAID, nonsteroidal anti-inflammatory drug; TNF, tumour necrosis factor. Adapted from http://www.spondylitis.org/physician_resources/guidelines.aspx.

More studies are needed to get a better idea of prognostic factors, which is also crucial for identifying patients who are in need of early, more aggressive therapy.

The use of TNF blockers in early non-radiographic axial SpA

As AS patients with a shorter disease duration respond better to TNF-blocker treatment and as there can be ongoing active inflammation in the SI joints and/or spine for some time before radiographic changes become visible, it is logical to question whether, and how well, active axial SpA patients with non-radiographic sacroiliitis respond to treatment with TNF blockers. If these patients were treated with adalimumab for 12 weeks an ASAS 40 response was achieved in 54% of patients versus 12% in the placebo group, an effect that was maintained over 1 year of treatment for the whole group after the placebo patients were also switched to adalimumab [95]. In the subgroup of patients with a disease duration of less than 3 years such a major response was achieved in 80% of patients. A similar result was reported for patients with early axial SpA with symptom duration of less than 3 years when treated with infliximab [98]. In this study a partial remission was achieved in 55%. Thus, treatment with a TNF blocker seems to be more effective the earlier the patients are treated. Preliminary results from these two studies indicate that most patients relapse if treatment is stopped. It remains to be seen whether long-lasting drug-free remission can be achieved if patients are treated even earlier.

The new classification criteria for axial SpA (see Figure 4.9, Chapter 4) now also cover this group of patients [7]. This is a very important first step for an extension of the label for TNF-blocker treatment from AS patients (normally fulfilling the modified New York criteria) to patients with non-radiographic axial SpA. Indeed, we were able recently to show that patients with non-radiographic axial SpA have the same level of disease activity and the same level of pain as patients with radiographic axial SpA (AS), and they therefore have a similar demand for effective treatment with TNF blockers if conventional treatment fails [9].

Other treatment options

Currently there are no other medical treatment options for AS patients. This creates a problem particularly in those patients who do not respond sufficiently to TNF blockers. Although there are now several other biologics that are effective in rheumatoid arthritis, such data are missing for AS. However, treatment trials with various biologics are currently ongoing or planned in AS.

Which instruments should be used for clinical record keeping?

The Bath Ankylosing Spondylitis Disease Activity Index (BASDAI) is a questionnaire filled in by the patient – covering fatigue, back pain, peripheral joint pain, pain of entheses and morning stiffness – and is normally used for the assessment of disease activity (Figure 6.26) [99]. It does not help to differentiate AS from other causes of back pain but gives a good estimate of the level of disease activity in an AS patient, if symptoms are caused by inflammation. In addition to the BASDAI, ASAS has proposed a core set for clinical record keeping which is shown in Figure 6.27 [100]. The functional index BASFI (Bath Ankylosing Spondylitis Functional Index) is shown in Figure 6.28 and Figures

3.3–3.7 (see Chapter 3) showed how to measure spinal mobility [101]. BASDAI and BASFI should be assessed about every 3–6 months and spinal mobility about every 6–12 months, depending on the level of disease activity and progression of the disease. These instruments have also been used as outcome parameters in clinical trials. A more detailed description is given in the recently published ASAS handbook on the assessment of spondyloarthritis [51].

Bath Ankylosing Spondylitis Disease Activity Index

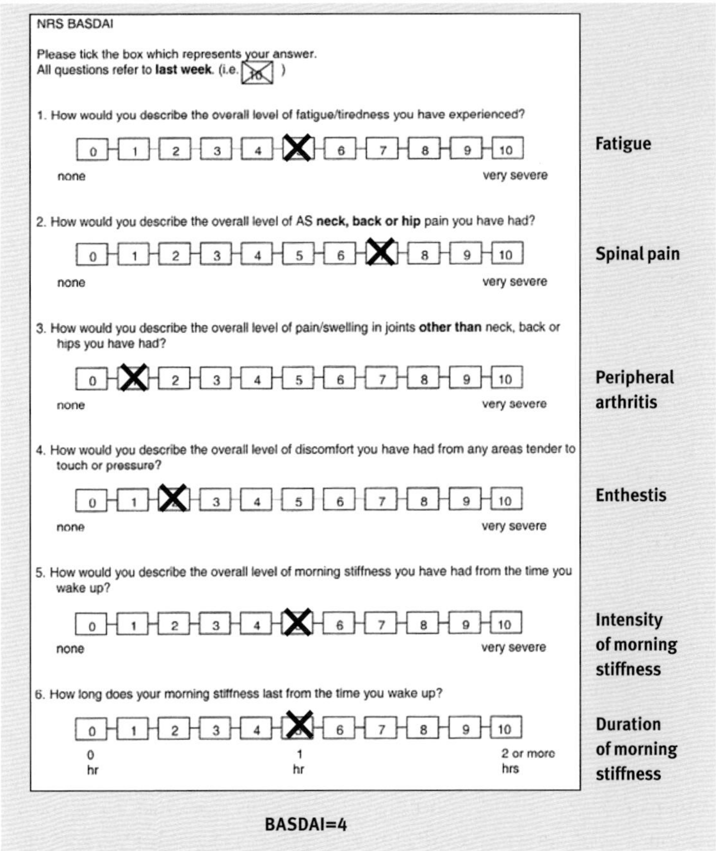

NRS BASDAI

Please tick the box which represents your answer.
All questions refer to **last week**. (i.e. [X])

1. How would you describe the overall level of fatigue/tiredness you have experienced?
0 1 2 3 4 5 6 7 8 9 10
none — very severe

2. How would you describe the overall level of AS **neck, back or hip** pain you have had?
0 1 2 3 4 5 6 7 8 9 10
none — very severe

3. How would you describe the overall level of pain/swelling in joints **other than** neck, back or hips you have had?
0 1 2 3 4 5 6 7 8 9 10
none — very severe

4. How would you describe the overall level of discomfort you have had from any areas tender to touch or pressure?
0 1 2 3 4 5 6 7 8 9 10
none — very severe

5. How would you describe the overall level of morning stiffness you have had from the time you wake up?
0 1 2 3 4 5 6 7 8 9 10
none — very severe

6. How long does your morning stiffness last from the time you wake up?
0 1 2 3 4 5 6 7 8 9 10
0 hr — 1 hr — 2 or more hrs

Figure 6.26 Bath Ankylosing Spondylitis Disease Activity Index. BASDAI, Bath Ankylosing Spondylitis Disease Activity Index. In the example above, the BASDAI=4. The BASDAI is calculated by adding the mean of questions 5 and 6, to the sum of questions 1–4, the total figure is then divided by 5. Adapted with permission from Garrett et al. [99].

ASAS core set for clinical record keeping

Domain	Instrument
1. Function	BASFI
2. Pain	NRS/VAS-last week-spine-at night-due to AS and NRS/VAS-last week-spine-due to AS
3. Spinal mobility	Chest expansion and modified Schober and occiput to wall and cervical rotation and (lateral spinal flexion or BASMI)
4. Patient global	NRS/VAS-global disease activity last week
5. Peripheral joints and entheses	Number of swollen joints (44 joint count) Validated enthesitis score, such as MASES, San Francisco and Berlin
6. Stiffness	NRS / VAS duration of morning stiffness -spine-last week
7. Acute phase reactants	Erythrocyte sedimentation rate
8. Fatigue	Fatigue question BASDAI

Figure 6.27 ASAS core set for clinical record keeping. AS, ankylosing spondylitis; BASDAI, Bath Ankylosing Spondylitis Disease Activity Index; BASFI, Bath Ankylosing Spondylitis Functional Index; BASMI, Bath Ankylosing Spondylitis Metrology Index; MASES, Maastricht Ankylosing Spondylitis Enthesitis Score; NRS, numerical rating scale; VAS, visual analogue scale. Reproduced with permission from van der Heijde et al. [100].

Bath Ankylosing Spondylitis Functional Index

Please indicate your level of ability with each of the following activities during the past week

All items scored on a 0–10 numerical rating scale* (0 = easy, 10 = impossible)

1.   Putting on your socks or tights without help or aids (eg, sock aid)

2.   Bending forward from the waist to pick up a pen from the floor without aid

3.   Reaching up to a high shelf without help or aids (eg, a helping hand)

4.   Getting up out of an armless dining room chair without using your hands or any other help

5.   Getting up off the floor without help from lying on your back

6.   Standing unsupported for 10 minutes without discomfort

7.   Climbing 12–15 steps without using a handrail or walking aid (one foot at each step)

8.   Looking over your shoulder without turning your body

9.   Doing physically demanding activities (eg, physiotherapy, exercises, gardening or sports)

10.   Doing a full days activities, whether it be at home or at work

The BASFI is the mean of 10 item-scores completed on a numerical rating scale

Figure 6.28 Bath Ankylosing Spondylitis Functional Index. BASFI, Bath Ankylosing Spondylitis Functional Index. *A visual analogue scale (0–100) can also be used. Adapted with permission from Calin et al. [101].

Chapter 7

Socioeconomic aspects of ankylosing spondylitis

Mainly as a result of the high costs for treatment with tumour necrosis factor (TNF) blockers the analysis of socioeconomic data for ankylosing spondylitis, as for other chronic diseases, has become of great interest. In these kinds of analyses direct and indirect costs caused by the disease are balanced against treatment costs, savings of direct and indirect costs, and gain in quality of life. Quality of life has been found to be equally reduced in patients with ankylosing spondylitis and in patients with rheumatoid arthritis, but healthcare costs were higher in rheumatoid arthritis [40]. An effort has been made to calculate the cost-effectiveness of the TNF-blocking agents infliximab and etanercept in the treatment of ankylosing spondylitis [102, 103]. Such a treatment seems to be cost-effective when the reduction of direct and indirect costs and the gain in quality of life are calculated against the drug costs, especially in patients with high disease activity and good response to treatment. However, future research is necessary to learn more about the natural course of the disease, prognostic factors and long-term effects of the treatment with TNF-blocking agents.

References

1. Braun J, Sieper J. Ankylosing spondylitis. Lancet 2007; 369:1379–90.
2. van der Linden S, Valkenburg HA, et al. Evaluation of diagnostic criteria for ankylosing spondylitis. A proposal for modification of the New York criteria. Arthritis Rheum 1984; 27:361–8.
3. Braun J, Bollow M, et al. Use of dynamic magnetic resonance imaging with fast imaging in the detection of early and advanced sacroiliitis in spondylarthropathy patients. Arthritis Rheum 1994; 37:1039–45.
4. Rudwaleit M, Khan MA, et al. The challenge of diagnosis and classification in early ankylosing spondylitis: do we need new criteria? Arthritis Rheum 2005; 52:1000–8.
5. Dougados M, van der Linden S, et al. The European Spondylarthropathy Study Group preliminary criteria for the classification of spondylarthropathy. Arthritis Rheum 1991; 34:1218–27.
6. Amor B, Dougados M, et al. [Criteria of the classification of spondylarthropathies]. Rev Rhum Mal Osteoartic 1990; 57: 85–9.
7. Rudwaleit M, van der Heijde D, et al. The development of Assessment of SpondyloArthritis international Society (ASAS) classification criteria for axial spondyloarthritis (Part II): validation and final selection. Ann Rheum Dis 2009; in press.
8. Feldtkeller E, Bruckel J, et al. Scientific contributions of ankylosing spondylitis patient advocacy groups. Curr opin Rheumatol 2000; 12: 239–47.
9. Rudwaleit M, Haibel H, et al. The early disease stage in axial spondyloarthritis. Results from the German spondyloarthritis inception cohort. Arthritis Rheum 2009; 60: 717–27.
10. Calin A, Fries JF. Striking prevalence of ankylosing spondylitis in 'healthy' w27 positive males and females. N Engl J Med 1975; 293:835–9.
11. van der Linden S, Valkenburg HA, et al. The risk of developing ankylosing spondylitis in HLA-B27 positive individuals: a comparison of relatives of spondylitis patients with the general population. Arthritis Rheum 1984; 27:241–9.
12. Braun J, Listing J, et al. Reply. Arthritis Rheum 2005; 52:4049–59.
13. Gran T, Husby G, et al. Prevalence of ankylosing spondylitis in males and females in a young middle aged population in Tromso, northern Norway. Ann Rheum Dis 1985; 44:359–67.
14. Gofton JP, Robinson HS, et al. Ankylosing spondylitis in a Canadian Indian population. Ann Rheum Dis 1966; 25:525–7.
15. Saraux A, Guillemin F, et al. Prevalence of spondyloarthropathies in France: 2001. Ann Rheum Dis 2005; 64:1431–5.
16. Guillemin F, Saraux A, et al. Prevalence of rheumatoid arthritis in France: 2001. Ann Rheum Dis 2005; 64:1427–30.
17. Adomaviciute D, Pileckyte M, et al. Prevalence survey of rheumatoid arthritis and spondyloarthropathy in Lithuania. Scand J Rheumatol 2008; 37:113–19.
18. Helmick CG, Felson DT, et al. Estimates of the prevalence of arthritis and other rheumatic conditions in the United States. Part I. Arthritis Rheum 2008; 58:15–25.

19. Sieper J, Rudwaleit M, et al. Concepts and epidemiology of spondyloarthritis. Best Pract Res Clin Rheumatol 2006; 20:401–17.

20. Brewerton DA, Hart FD, et al. Ankylosing spondylitis and HLA-27. Lancet 1973; i: 904–7.

21. Sieper J, Braun J, et al. Report on the fourth international workshop on reactive arthritis. Arthritis Rheum 2000; 43:720–34.

22. Maksymowych WP. Ankylosing spondylitis -- at the interface of bone and cartilage. J Rheumatol 2000; 27:2295–301.

23. Appel H, Kuhne M, et al. Immunohistochemical analysis of hip arthritis in ankylosing spondylitis: evaluation of the bone-cartilage interface and subchondral bone marrow. Arthritis Rheum 2006; 54:1805–13.

24. Sieper J, Appel H, et al. Critical appraisal of assessment of structural damage in ankylosing spondylitis: implications for treatment outcomes. Arthritis Rheum 2008; 58:649–56.

25. Appel H, Sieper J. Spondyloarthritis at the crossroads of imaging, pathology, and structural damage in the era of biologics. Curr Rheumatol Rep 2008;10:356–63.

26. Maksymowych WP, Chiowchanwisawakit P, et al. Inflammatory lesions of the spine on magnetic resonance imaging predict the development of new syndesmophytes in ankylosing spondylitis: evidence of a relationship between inflammation and new bone formation. Arthritis Rheum 2009; 60:93–102.

27. Brown MA, Kennedy LG, et al. Susceptibility to ankylosing spondylitis in twins: the role of genes, HLA, and the environment. Arthritis Rheum 1997; 40:1823–8.

28. Burton PR, Clayton DG, et al. Association scan of 14,500 nonsynonymous SNPs in four diseases identifies autoimmunity variants. Nat Genet 2007; 39:1329–37.

29. Brown MA, Laval SH, et al. Recurrence risk modelling of the genetic susceptibility to ankylosing spondylitis. Ann Rheum Dis 2000; 59:883–6.

30. Calin A, Porta J, et al. Clinical history as a screening test for ankylosing spondylitis. JAMA 1977; 237:2613–4.

31. Sieper J, van der Heijde D, et al. New criteria for inflammatory back pain in patients with chronic back pain - a real patient exercise of the Assessment in SpondyloArthritis international Society (ASAS). Ann Rheum Dis 2009; In press.

32. Rudwaleit M, Metter A, et al. Inflammatory back pain in ankylosing spondylitis: a reassessment of the clinical history for application as classification and diagnostic criteria. Arthritis Rheum 2006; 54:569–78.

33. Rudwaleit M, van der Heijde D, et al. How to diagnose axial spondyloarthritis early. Ann Rheum Dis 2004; 63:535–43.

34. Baraliakos X, Listing J, et al. Progression of radiographic damage in patients with ankylosing spondylitis: defining the central role of syndesmophytes. Ann Rheum Dis 2007; 66: 910–5.

35. Landewe R, Dougados M, et al. Physical function in ankylosing spondylitis is independently determined by both disease activity and radiographic damage of the spine. Ann Rheum Dis 2008; in press.

36. Vander Cruyssen B, Ribbens C, et al. The epidemiology of ankylosing spondylitis and the commencement of anti-TNF therapy in daily rheumatology practice. Ann Rheum Dis 2007; 66:1072–7.

37. McGonagle D, Gibbon W, et al. Characteristic magnetic resonance imaging entheseal changes of knee synovitis in spondylarthropathy. Arthritis Rheum 1998; 41:694–700.

38. Lambert RG, Dhillon SS, et al. High prevalence of symptomatic enthesiopathy of the shoulder in ankylosing spondylitis: deltoid origin involvement constitutes a hallmark of disease. Arthritis Rheum 2004; 51:681–90.

39. Zeboulon N, Dougados M, et al. Prevalence and characteristics of uveitis in the spondyloarthropathies: a systematic literature review. Ann Rheum Dis 2008; 67:955–9.

40. Verstappen SM, Jacobs JW, et al. Utility and direct costs: ankylosing spondylitis compared with rheumatoid arthritis. Ann Rheum Dis 2007; 66:727–31.

41. Burgos-Vargas R, Vazquez-Mellado J. The early clinical recognition of juvenile-onset ankylosing spondylitis and its differentiation from juvenile rheumatoid arthritis. Arthritis Rheum 1995; 38:835–44.

42. Bennett PH, Burch TA (eds.). Population studies of the rheumatic diseases. Amsterdam: Excerpta Medica Foundation, International Congress Series 1966, 148: 456–7.

43. Rudwaleit M, Jurik AG, et al. The Assessment in SpondyloArthritis international Society (ASAS) definition of sacroiliitis on magnetic resonance imaging (MRI) – a consensual approach. Ann Rheum Dis 2009; in press.

44. Bennett AN, McGonagle D, et al. Severity of baseline magnetic resonance imaging-evident sacroiliitis and HLA-B27 status in early inflammatory back pain predict radiographically evident ankylosing spondylitis at eight years. Arthritis Rheum 2008; 58: 3413–18.

45. Underwood MR, Dawes P. Inflammatory back pain in primary care. Br J Rheumatol 1995; 34:1074–7.

46. Sieper J, Rudwaleit M. Early referral recommendations for ankylosing spondylitis (including pre-radiographic and radiographic forms) in primary care. Ann Rheum Dis 2005; 64:659–63.

47. Brandt HC, Spiller I, et al. Performance of referral recommendations in patients with chronic back pain and suspected axial spondyloarthritis. Ann Rheum Dis 2007; 66:1479–84.

48. Baraliakos X, Listing J, et al. Radiographic progression in patients with ankylosing spondylitis after 2 years of treatment with the tumor necrosis factor and antibody infliximab. Ann Rheum Dis 2005; 64:1462–1466.

49. Vosse D, Landewe R, et al. Ankylosing spondylitis and the risk of fracture: results from a large primary care-based nested case control study. Ann Rheum Dis 2008; in press.

50. Sieper J. Management of ankylosing spondylitis. In: Rheumatology, 4th edition. Edited by MC Hochberg, AJ Silman, et al. London: Mosby, 2008; 1159.

51. Sieper J, Rudwaleit M, et al. The Assessment of SpondyloArthritis international Society (ASAS) handbook: a guide to assess spondyloarthritis. Ann Rheum Dis 2009; in press.

52. Braun J, Bollow M, et al. Radiologic diagnosis and pathology of the spondyloarthropathies. Rheum Dis Clin North Am 1998; 24:697–735.

53. Song IH, Carrasco-Fernandez J, et al. The diagnostic value of scintigraphy in assessing sacroiliitis in ankylosing spondylitis: a systematic literature research. Ann Rheum Dis 2008; 67:1535–40.

54. Zochling J, van der Heijde D, et al. ASAS/EULAR recommendations for the management of ankylosing spondylitis. Ann Rheum Dis 2006; 65:442–52.

55. Anderson JJ, Baron G, et al. Ankylosing spondylitis assessment group preliminary definition of short-term improvement in ankylosing spondylitis. Arthritis Rheum 2001; 44:1876–86.

56. Song IH, Poddubnyy DA, et al. Benefits and risks of ankylosing spondylitis treatment with nonsteroidal anti-inflammatory drugs. Arthritis Rheum 2008; 58:929–38.

57. Amor B, Dougados M, et al. Are classification criteria for spondylarthropathy useful as diagnostic criteria? Rev Rheum Engl Ed 1995; 62:10–15.

58. Gossec L, Dougados M, et al. Dissemination and evaluation of the ASAS/EULAR recommendations for the management of ankylosing spondylitis: results of a study among 1507 rheumatologists. Ann Rheum Dis 2008; 67:782–8.

59. Wanders A, Heijde D, et al. Nonsteroidal anti-inflammatory drugs reduce radiographic progression in patients with ankylosing spondylitis: a randomized clinical trial. Arthritis Rheum 2005; 52:1756–65.

60. Braun J, Bollow M, et al. Computed tomography guided corticosteroid injection of the sacroiliac joint in patients with spondyloarthropathy with sacroiliitis: clinical outcome and followup by dynamic magnetic resonance imaging. J Rheumatol 1996; 23:659–64.

61. Haibel H, Rudwaleit M, et al. Open label trial of anakinra in active ankylosing spondylitis over 24 weeks. Ann Rheum Dis 2005; 64:296–8.

62. Haibel H, M Rudwaleit, et al. Six months open label trial of leflunomide in active ankylosing spondylitis. Ann Rheum Dis 2005; 64:124–6.

63. Haibel H, Brandt HC, et al. No efficacy of subcutaneous methotrexate in active ankylosing spondylitis: a 16-week open-label trial. Ann Rheum Dis 2007; 66:419–21.

64. Dougados M, van der Linden S, et al. Sulfasalazine in the treatment of spondylarthropathy. A randomized, multicenter, double-blind, placebo-controlled study. Arthritis Rheum 1995; 38:618–27.

65. Braun J, Zochling J, et al. Efficacy of sulfasalazine in patients with inflammatory back pain due to undifferentiated spondyloarthritis and early ankylosing spondylitis: a multicentre randomised controlled trial. Ann Rheum Dis 2006; 65:1147–53.

66. Haibel H, Brandt HC, et al. No efficacy of subcutaneous methotrexate in active ankylosing spondylitis: a 16-week open-label trial. Ann Rheum Dis 2007; 66:419–21.

67. Brandt J, Listing J, et al. Development and preselection of criteria for short term improvement after anti-TNF alpha treatment in ankylosing spondylitis. Ann Rheum Dis 2004; 63:1438–44.

68. van der Heijde D, Dijkmans B, et al. Efficacy and safety of infliximab in patients with ankylosing spondylitis: results of a randomized, placebo-controlled trial (ASSERT). Arthritis Rheum 2005; 52:582–91.

69. van der Heijde D, Kivitz A, et al. Adalimumab therapy results in significant reduction of signs and symptoms in subjects with ankylosing spondylitis: the ATLAS trial. Arthritis Rheum 2006; 54 2136–46.

70. Davis JC, van der Heijde DM, et al. Sustained durability and tolerability of etanercept in ankylosing spondylitis for 96 weeks. Ann Rheum Dis 2005; 64:1557–62.

71. Braun J, Brandt J, et al. Treatment of active ankylosing spondylitis with infliximab: a randomised controlled multicentre trial. Lancet 2002; 359:1187–93.

72. Davis JC Jr, Van Der Heijde D, et al. Recombinant human tumor necrosis factor receptor (etanercept) for treating ankylosing spondylitis: a randomized, controlled trial. Arthritis Rheum 2003; 48:3230–6.

73. van der Heijde D, Lie E, et al. The ASDAS is a highly discriminatory ASAS-endorsed disease activity score in patients with ankylosing spondylitis. Ann Rheum Dis 2008; in press.

74. Braun J, Landewe R, et al. Major reduction in spinal inflammation in patients with ankylosing spondylitis after treatment with infliximab: results of a multicenter, randomized, double-blind, placebo-controlled magnetic resonance imaging study. Arthritis Rheum 2006; 54:1646–52.

75. Rudwaleit M, Baraliakos X, et al. Magnetic resonance imaging of the spine and the sacroiliac joints in ankylosing spondylitis and undifferentiated spondyloarthritis during treatment with etanercept. Ann Rheum Dis 2005; 64:1305–10.

76. Lambert RG, Salonen D, et al. Adalimumab significantly reduces both spinal and sacroiliac joint inflammation in patients with ankylosing spondylitis: a multicenter, randomized, double-blind, placebo-controlled study. Arthritis Rheum 2007; 56:4005–14.

77. Sieper J, Baraliakos X, et al. Persistent reduction of spinal inflammation as assessed by magnetic resonance imaging in patients with ankylosing spondylitis after 2 yrs of treatment with the anti-tumour necrosis factor agent infliximab. Rheumatology (Oxford) 2005; 44:1525–30.

78. Heiberg MS, Nordvag BY, et al. The comparative effectiveness of tumor necrosis factor-blocking agents in patients with rheumatoid arthritis and patients with ankylosing spondylitis: a six-month, longitudinal, observational, multicenter study. Arthritis Rheum 2005; 52:2506–12.

79. Braun J, Deodhar A, et al. Efficacy and safety of infliximab in patients with ankylosing spondylitis over a two-year period. Arthritis Rheum 2008; 59:1270–8.

80. van der Heijde D, Landewe R, et al. Radiographic findings following two years of infliximab therapy in patients with ankylosing spondylitis. Arthritis Rheum 2008; 58:3063–70.

81. van der Heijde D, Landewe R, et al. Radiographic progression of ankylosing spondylitis after up to two years of treatment with etanercept. Arthritis Rheum 2008; 58:1324–31.

82. Braun J, Sieper J. What is the most important outcome parameter in ankylosing spondylitis? Rheumatology (Oxford) 2008; 47:1738–40.

83. Breban M, Ravaud P, et al. Maintenance of infliximab treatment in ankylosing spondylitis: results of a one-year randomized controlled trial comparing systematic versus on-demand treatment. Arthritis Rheum 2008; 58: 88–97.

84. Li EK, Griffith JF, et al. Short-term efficacy of combination methotrexate and infliximab in patients with ankylosing spondylitis: a clinical and magnetic resonance imaging correlation. Rheumatology (Oxford) 2008; 47:1358–63.

85. Braun J, Baraliakos X, et al. Differences in the incidence of flares or new onset of inflammatory bowel diseases in patients with ankylosing spondylitis exposed to therapy with anti-tumor necrosis factor alpha agents. Arthritis Rheum 2007; 57:639–47.

86. van der Heijde D, Schiff MH, et al. Adalimumab effectiveness for the treatment of ankylosing spondylitis is maintained for up to 2 years: long-term results from the ATLAS trial. Ann Rheum Dis 2008; in press.

87. Braun J, Baraliakos X, et al. Decreased incidence of anterior uveitis in patients with ankylosing spondylitis treated with the anti-tumor necrosis factor agents infliximab and etanercept. Arthritis Rheum 2005; 52:2447–51.

88. Rudwaleit M, Rodevand E, et al. Adalimumab effectively reduces the rate of anterior uveitis flares in patients with active ankylosing spondylitis: results of a prospective open-label study. Ann Rheum Dis 2008; in press.

89. Braun J, Baraliakos X, et al. Persistent clinical efficacy and safety of anti-tumour necrosis factor alpha therapy with infliximab in patients with ankylosing spondylitis over 5 years: evidence for different types of response. Ann Rheum Dis 2008; 67; 340–5.

90. Baraliakos X, Listing J, et al. Persistent clinical efficacy and safety of infliximab in patients with ankylosing spondylitis over 7 years – evidence for different response to anti-TNF-A therapy. Presented at: EULAR, the Annual European Congress of Rheumatology, Paris, France; June 11–14, 2008; FR10290.

91. Keat A, Barkham N, et al. BSR guidelines for prescribing TNF-alpha blockers in adults with ankylosing spondylitis. Report of a working party of the British Society for Rheumatology. Rheumatology (Oxford) 2005; 44:939–47.

92. Maksymowych WP, Gladman D, et al. The Canadian Rheumatology Association/ Spondyloarthritis Research Consortium of Canada treatment recommendations for the management of spondyloarthritis: a national multidisciplinary stakeholder project. J Rheumatol 2007; 34:2273–84.

93. Braun J, Davis J, et al. ASAS Working Group. First update of the international ASAS consensus statement for the use of anti-TNF agents in patients with ankylosing spondylitis. Ann Rheum Dis 2006; 65:316–20.

94. Rudwaleit M, Listing J, et al. Prediction of a major clinical response (BASDAI 50) to tumour necrosis factor alpha blockers in ankylosing spondylitis. Ann Rheum Dis 2004; 63:665–70.

95. Haibel H, Rudwaleit M, et al. Efficacy of adalimumab in the treatment of axial spondylarthritis without radiographically defined sacroiliitis: results of a twelve-week randomized, double-blind, placebo-controlled trial followed by an open-label extension up to week fifty-two. Arthritis Rheum 2008; 58:1981–91.

96. Rudwaleit M, Schwarzlose S, et al. MRI in predicting a major clinical response to anti-tumour necrosis factor treatment in ankylosing spondylitis. Ann Rheum Dis 2008; 67:1276–81.

97. Amor B, Santos RS, et al. Predictive factors for the longterm outcome of spondyloarthropathies. J Rheumatol 1994; 21:1883–7.

98. Barkham N, Keen H, et al. A randomised controlled trial of infliximab shows clinical and MRI efficacy in patients with HLA-B27 positive very early ankylosing spondylitis. Presented at: 71st annual scientific meeting of the American College of Rheumatology. Boston, Massachusetts; November 6–11, 2007; (Abstract #L11).

99. Garrett S, Jenkinson T, et al. A new approach to defining disease status in ankylosing spondylitis: the Bath Ankylosing Spondylitis Disease Activity Index. J Rheumatol 1994; 21:2286–91.

100. van der Heijde D, Calin A, et al. Selection of instruments in the core set for DC-ART, SMARD, physical therapy, and clinical record keeping in ankylosing spondylitis. Progress report of the ASAS Working Group. Assessments in Ankylosing Spondylitis. J Rheumatol 1999; 26:951–4.

101. Calin A, Garrett S, et al. A new approach to defining functional ability in ankylosing spondylitis: the development of the Bath Ankylosing Spondylitis Functional Index. J Rheumatol 1994; 21:2281–5.

102. Boonen A, van der Heijde D, et al. Markov model into the cost-utility over five years of etanercept and infliximab compared with usual care in patients with active ankylosing spondylitis. Ann Rheum Dis 2006; 65:201–8.

103. Kobelt G, Sobocki P, et al. The cost-effectiveness of infliximab in the treatment of ankylosing spondylitis in Spain. Comparison of clinical trial and clinical practice data. Scand J Rheumatol 2008; 37:62–71.